To: My new best friend, Claud Brockett
Given in memory of Merlin Brockett
Feb 2, 2005
Joe Parks

Donkey Foaling Manual

By Bonnie R. Gross

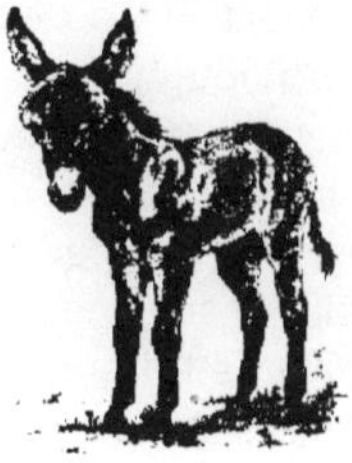

ISBN 0-9658547-3-6

Library of Congress Catalog Card Number: 99-091700

Author: Bonnie R. Gross

Publisher: Miniature Donkey Talk, Inc.
1338 Hughes Shop Road, Westminster, Maryland 21158
Telephone 410-875-0118

DISCLAIMER: The suggestions, recommendations and advice in this book are written in the hope that readers will accept the information as a guide and apply them accordingly. Although every effort has been made to present accurate, up-to-date information, it should be understood that the results of medical treatments depend upon many factors, including proper diagnosis and individual conditions. Therefore, neither the Author nor the Publisher assumes responsibility for and makes no warranty with respect to results that may be obtained from the procedures herein. Neither the Author nor the Publisher shall be liable to any person for damage resulting from reliance on any information contained in this book. To ensure the reader's understanding of some technical descriptions offered in this book, brand names have been used as examples of particular substances or equipment. However, the use of a particular brand name is not intended to imply an endorsement of any particular product. Each reader should contact their own veterinarian and follow their advice before giving any medical treatment to their animals.

Dedicated to all Miniature Donkeys in the hope that your human friends can assist in bringing your foals into the world healthier and happier.

Bonnie Gross
Miniature Donkey Talk Magazine

CONTENTS

Chapter 1: Breeding Donkeys

Chapter 2: The Pregnant Jennet

Chapter 3: Getting Ready For The Foal

Chapter 4: The Foaling Process

Chapter 5: Jennet Aftercare

Chapter 6: The Newborn

Chapter 7: Foal Illness and Disease

Chapter 8: Weanlings

Chapter 9: Jacks

Chapter 10: Miscellaneous Health Care

Chapter 11: Buying, Selling, Marketing

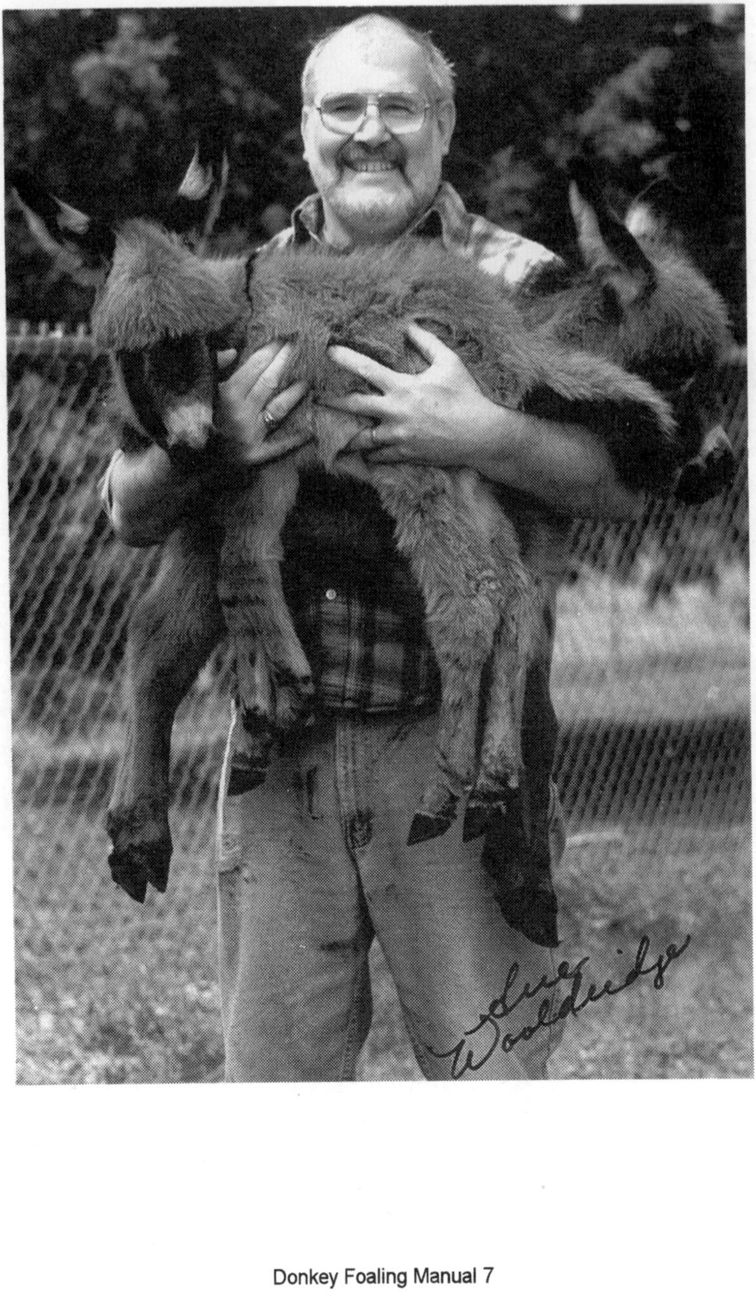

Chapter 1

Breeding Donkeys

Introduction to the Miniature Donkey

Life Span:
With proper lifelong care, 25-40 years
Height:
36" or under (IMDR Class A Registry), 38" or under (IMDR Class B Registry)
Weight:
200 to 450 pounds
Males:
Any age male is called a Jack
Females:
Any age female is called a Jennet

HISTORY:

Miniature donkeys are native to the Mediterranean islands of Sicily and Sardinia. It is difficult to import them now because 1) The quality of donkey left in Sicily and Sardinia is not good, and, 2) It is very difficult to pass the tests given by quarantine stations at the Dept. of Agriculture. However, this writer purchased two donkeys imported into this country from Sicily 10 years ago so the task is not impossible, just improbable. Miniature Donkeys have not been bred down in size per se. The 25-30 Miniature Donkeys originally imported into the U.S. were between the sizes of 32" and 38" with the majority of them being in the 35"-37" size range. Over the years, breeders have concentrated more on the 32"-33" size and today your most desirable and well-conformed donkeys are from 31" to 35". The word "miniature" usually refers to animals that have been bred-down in size, so keep in mind that 'miniature donkeys' are simply diminutive and not bred down such is the case of many other 'miniature' animals.

COLOR:

The most prevalent color for Miniature Donkeys is gray-dun which consists of a gray colored body, light colored nose - or dark colored nose -, light colored belly and inside legs, with a dark color dorsal stripe down the back and over the shoulders. The dorsal stripe is known as the donkeys cross. There are variations of this gray-dun from dark to light. As with most animals, donkeys can range in color from black to white and everything in between. True blacks are extremely rare with black/browns (not quite black) being more common. There are chestnut/sorrels which are various shades of reddish brown. There are also white donkeys and "spotted" donkeys. Some people refer to spotted as "pinto" and this really boils down to semantics. Spotted or pintos are generally gray or brown and white. There are also various colors of roans. Roan coloring is black, brown, gray hairs intermingled with white hairs. Donkeys do not breed true to color. Since gray-dun is by far the predominant gene, you can breed black to black and get gray-dun, spotted to spotted and get gray-dun, etc. Never knowing what color foal will be produced is part of the excitement of having foals. Colors other than the typical gray-dun make the donkey more exotic looking therefore increases their price.

REPRODUCTION:

Jennets can become fertile at one year of age but if bred, make very poor mothers and usually reject their foals. Jennets can be considered for breeding after the age of two or 2-1/2 years depending on their overall physical and mental maturity. Miniature Donkeys, on average, carry a foal for 12 months. Average Gestation: 11 months, 3 weeks, 5 days. (Unlike other animals, donkeys can carry their foals from 11 months to 13 months.) Most are not rebred until their second heat cycle, some 30 odd days after foaling. Some jennets will not conceive until their foal is weaned. Taking all into consideration, the average jennet produces one offspring every 13 to 14 months.

Jacks (males) can be fertile at one year of age but generally wait until 16 to 18 months. The famed herd sire "Charlie Bandito" owned by Pheasant Meadow Farm in Maryland, produced his first offspring at the age of 12 months and his first son, "Guido Bandito" produced his first offspring at the age of 12-1/2 months. Some smaller sized jacks - 31" and under - may not show an interest in breeding until they are two years old. Jacks inherit much of their overall fertility and libido from their sires. Twinning in Miniature Donkeys is rare. Birth weights are generally between 18 and 25 pounds. jennets between the size of 33" and 38" usually have an easy time foaling. Smaller jennets may need human intervention.

HEALTH CARE:

Miniature Donkeys are very healthy animals. They require the same yearly vaccinations as horses. They should also be dewormed, with an equine dewormer, at a minimum of three times per year, preferably six times per year. They require the same hoof care as horses and should be trimmed at least three or four times per year. See the book *Caring For Your Miniature*

FEEDING:

Donkeys can survive on good quality hay alone. A good hay to feed donkeys is a mixture of 1/4 alfalfa and 3/4 grass. Pure alfalfa is too rich a feed for Miniature Donkeys and does not set well with their digestive systems. They can also become extremely fat. With severe droughts often occurring in different parts of the country, sometimes only poor quality hay is available and in this case, donkeys should be supplemented with a 10-12% protein equine sweet feed. Donkeys are termed as "easy keepers" meaning they utilize their feed very efficiently and you must be careful that they do not get fat. Fat donkeys will develop a "crest" - or fat roll - on their necks that will be there for life once it develops.

Limited acreage can go hand in hand with Miniature Donkeys. You could easily keep 10 donkeys on an acre of land. This however doesn't mean they could live off pasture grasses. It does mean they could live comfortably being fed hay year round. You basically need a pasture large enough for them to run and play in to receive enough exercise for them to remain healthy.

PERSONALITY:

The first and foremost attraction to Miniature Donkeys is their loving personalities. They demand attention! They form close attachments to their owners and to other donkeys. Donkeys are herd animals and one lone donkey is a very lonely donkey. Because of their laid-back, easy going personalities, they make wonderful pets for children, the handicapped and the elderly. I do not recommend that you buy an ungelded adult jack as a pet. Even though the donkey's nature is to be much less nervous and tense than an ungelded horse, you cannot remove his basic instincts. You can buy an ungelded jack foal and at approximately one year of age, have him gelded making him safe around seniors and children.

DONKEY COMMUNICATION:

Donkeys communicate with their human owners and with other donkeys by "braying", also more commonly known as a hee-haw. Every donkey has their own style of braying with some sounding quite comical. They range from barely being audible to a loud thunderous bray. Donkeys develop schedules and if you are late in feeding, you will hear about it! Jacks pastured apart from their jennets, will call to them several times a day. On the whole, donkeys are very quiet animals.

COST:

Prices on donkeys vary greatly depending on the region of the country and the quality of the animal. Pet jacks are the most economical. Breeding age jennets or bred jennets are the most expensive.

CONFORMATION:

Every breeder has their own idea of what they want to breed for. This is their privilege and their right as a breeder. There are miniature donkeys that are compact with a draft type build and other donkeys with slender more leggy builds. The International Miniature Donkey Registry has Breed Standards© for Miniature Donkeys (no charge) which are well worth reading.

Most people do not realize just how very important the conformation of their breeding jack is. A jack will determine 50% of the conformation of the foal. Not all jacks carry this strong conformation gene, however, if you desire to begin a breeding operation, your jack should be your most important purchase. When looking at breeding age jennets, smaller is not necessarily better! You want to keep the majority of your breeding jennets between the sizes of 32" to 36" and a breeding jack 30" to 33". The original donkeys brought into this country were between the sizes of 32" and 38". *The International Miniature Donkey Registry* in Maryland has a Class A - donkeys up to 36" and a Class B for donkeys 36+" to 38". jennets under the height of 32" may have foaling (birthing) problems with their first foal.

Four serious conformation defects you want to avoid when buying donkeys you intend to use for breeding purposes are extreme parrot mouth or monkey mouth, turned out front legs and cow-hocks. Parrot and monkey mouths are where the top or bottom teeth protrude out further than 1/4" from the opposite set of teeth. As an added note, I have personally looked into the mouths of hundreds of donkeys and can honestly say that many, many of donkeys have slight over or underbites of 1/16 to 1/4 inch. Many donkeys stand slightly cowhocked. You simply cannot compare the stature of a donkey to a horse and will do a donkey injustice if you do so. Severely cowhocked hind legs are a definite conformation defect and these donkeys should be avoided when you are purchasing breeding stock.

REGISTERED OR UNREGISTERED??

The International Miniature Donkey Registry in Maryland is a graded registry. If your intended purchase carries IMDR registration papers and that donkey has been graded (rated) by IMDR, and has achieved a Two or Three Star Rating, you can be certain that you are purchasing a quality animal. Even if the donkey only has a "standard certificate", it also means that the donkey has been reviewed by professionals at IMDR. If the registration paper does not say "pet quality" than it is in fact a breeding quality donkey. Never dismiss a donkey simply because it does not have an extended pedigree. Also, do not dismiss a donkey if it is not registered. Inspect your intended purchases closely, check their teeth and conformation, and make your decisions based on the quality of each individual animal.

AGE:

With life long proper care, donkeys can live well into their 30's (although I personally had a jennet live to 47 years of age) and jennets can produce foals into their early 20's. Older jennets are normally wonderful mothers and fantastic baby sitters to put in with foals being weaned.

HEIGHT:

Desirable heights of Miniature Donkeys will vary with almost every person you talk to. I suggest that people purchase jennets to be used for breeding be between the height of 32" to 36". The International Miniature Donkey Registry has a class B for sizes 36+" to 38" for original foundation stock donkeys. jennets between the size of 33" to 38" tend to have better conformation and an easier time of foaling than do smaller jennets. When buying jacks, again pay particular attention to conformation first, size second. I can assure you that Grandparents can play a large role in the conformation, coloring and height of a foal.

WHERE TO BUY:

Before buying any breed of animal you should do your homework and have an idea of what you are looking for. Hundreds of breeders advertise in *Miniature Donkey Talk Magazine* and will be happy to talk to you and share with you their experiences in raising and breeding Miniature Donkeys. We encourage you to contact us at the magazine or any of our advertisers to help you with your questions.

GUARD DONKEYS:

There is a big misconception that ALL donkeys make excellent guard animals. Not all donkeys make good guard animals. A jack that has not been gelded should never be used. There is only a 50/50 chance that a jennet or gelded jack will make a good guard donkey. It all depends on the donkey's personality and temperament. This goes for all sized donkeys. If you purchase a donkey from a breeder to use specifically for a guard animal, you should have arrangements with the breeder that if the donkey does not work out, you can return the donkey. Most people want guard donkeys as protection against coyotes or dogs. Not all donkeys hate dogs. Again, never assume that all donkeys are good guardian animals.

NOTE: See "Most Common Newbie Questions" at the back of this book.

Genotype Meet Phenotype

You may have heard the breeder who has a stallion (who happens to have the world's most crooked set of hocks) say that the animal should be evaluated on his beautiful head. "Every equine has his *faults,* and it doesn't matter that this one has crooked hocks. His full brother was a champion. It just stands to reason that he has greatness hidden away in his genes!"

A breeder who believes that a pedigree is all he needs to get a good idea of a stallion's "genetics" can get so caught up in pedigree study that he is oblivious to the animal he actually owns. When an owner's loyalty and desire to promote a particular stallion is combined with an over-fascination with pedigree study, breeding good equine can get lost in the shuffle.

Likewise, when a breeder begins to conceive of individual equine as merely representatives or variations of the stream of genetic inheritance called a bloodline, he can easily excuse structural or biochemical defects in individuals - for he believes that individuals are less important than the bloodline considered as a whole. Such breeders are very reluctant to cull. They contend that any individual in their bloodline is as good as any other; after all, the equine "carries good genes." Thus, they hope to obtain individuals of superior phenotype from whatever pedigreed stock they have, under whatever environmental conditions exist on their particular breeding farms.

Breeding programs lose ground when breeders begin to act as if they knew exactly how genes produced the equine standing in front of them (the phenotype). *Both genetic and* environmental factors determine *phenotype,* and sorting out the contribution of each is difficult. For example, breeders dread seeing foals with crooked legs - it not only means present and future problems, but it leaves the lingering doubt: did the farm's champion stallion pass that on? Or is the feeding program to blame? The different effects of genes and environment can be distinguished - but a program of progeny testing under uniform environmental conditions is required.
Exactly what is phenotype, then, and how is it different from genotype? Phenotype is defined as "how an animal looks".

Genotype is "the genetic constitution underlying physical appearance."

Thus, genotype seems to be an invisible black box which somehow determines the presence of traits that are visible in the phenotype.

To breeders, who can only see and measure the animal from the outside, the concept of a "gene" always has been, and must be, hypothetical.

For the equine breeder, there is only one useful plan: pay attention to the phenotype. And when you hear someone claiming that a stallion has greatness hidden in his genes, be like the folks from Missouri - say "show me!"

Watch Words

***Bloodline**:* A group of animals related to each other "by blood" - that is, they can all be traced back to only a few ancestors. Because of this, members of a bloodline "sample" only the genes which were present in those ancestors. Thus, on the average, more identical combinations of genes occur in any two members of a bloodline than in any two equine selected at random.

***Gene pool**:* The sum total of all the genes in a population of animals. The population can be on any scale - all the individuals registered as members of a particular breed, all the members of a particular bloodline or one broodmare band. An individual animal does not have a "gene pool" -an individual has a genotype.

***Heritability**:* That portion of the individual's phenotype which is due to the effect of his genes. A heritability estimate is expressed as a percentage. When this percentage is subtracted from 100, it gives an estimate of the environment's effect on the phenotype.

When an owner's loyalty to a particular stallion is combined with an over fascination with pedigree study, breeding good equine can get lost in the shuffle.

Reference: Written by Debbie Bennett, PhD

Prostaglandins: *Their Use and Function*

These are the new wonder drugs of the last few years in equine reproduction. Prostaglandin F2 alpha is used for treating dysfunctions of the reproductive cycle in mares and jennets. The drug is given to mares and jennets who do not come into visible heat and are not pregnant or who come into heat erratically. It can be used to bring a jennet in shortly after she has gone out of foal heat so that instead of waiting 21 to 25 days for the second heat, she may be bred about 15 days after she foals. This can be extremely detrimental to the reproductive tract that has not had enough time to heal after giving birth. It can be used to shorten the time between heat cycles when a jennet is missed or too many jennets are booked to the jack at the same time.

Prostaglandins are used in jennets who have too long a time between heat cycles. They bring the jennet back into heat and allow her to be bred sooner than her own hormones allow. They may be given for diagnostic purposes to problem jennets to see if they can be stimulated to come into a normal heat at all. These drugs can also be used to synchronize heat cycles among a number of jennets so that they will foal within a short period (for management reasons).

These drugs may also be used to abort early pregnancies, such as a jennet who is bred who should not have been covered or her pregnancy has been diagnosed as being twins. One dose may not do the job; it may be necessary to give it two or three days in a row. When abortion is produced in this way, the jennet may not come into a normal heat for several months.

Prostin is one of the drugs most commonly used and it should be used in accordance with the label directions. Prostaglandins only work on about 1/4 of the mares and jennets to whom they are given. The others often have hormone imbalances or an ovarian dysfunction so that they cannot respond. Most jennets show signs of heat within 3 to 7 days after treatment. This is generally a fertile heat and the mare or jennet can be bred at this time. Mild, transient side effects may occur with the drug. These are generally not severe enough to be treated. Most jennets will show signs of sweating and general nervousness. Most jennets show signs of heat with one treatment. A few will require two or three treatments.

While these drugs can work wonders in some cases, they are by no means a cure-all. If the jennet does not have the ability to ovulate or has other abnormalities, they will not work at all. Jennets who will not come into heat should be checked by your veterinarian to determine if they are doing so silently or if their ovaries are simply not functioning so that they cannot respond to the prostaglandin. Many jennets will have "silent heats", or show no signs of heat towards a jack, until their foals are several months old.

Prostaglandins are potent hormones. The reality of the changing hormonal concentrations in the body of an equine relative to changes in her sexual behavior during the estrous cycle is a complex interaction, not just a simple relationship of cause and effect. Changing the level of hormones in the body by artificial means can never, therefore, be simplistic. Administering one hormone at any given time may be likened to increasing one ingredient of a cake without reference to the other ingredients. When we give hormones to an equine much of the effect depends on the makeup or state of the jennet at the start of the treatment.

Since prostaglandins are potent hormones, they are not to be spilled on your skin while giving injections. Some labeling also advises against their being handled by pregnant women or people with asthma. They are not terribly dangerous drugs, but should be handled with respect. For donkeys, Estrumate is the drug of choice.

Hand Breeding Verses Pasture Breeding

Many new owners have no idea how to go about the breeding process - to keep a jack in with jennets full time or to separate the jack in his own pasture and hand breed when the jennet comes in heat.

Pasture Breeding: Pasture breeding is of course the 'easy way out'. The jack lives full time with the jennets and breeds them when they come in heat. However, there are many negatives to pasture breeding. 1. You seldom have an accurate breeding date. 2. Jacks will start breeding the jennet when she first comes into heat greatly depleting his sperm count as jennets generally do not produce an egg to be fertilized until the 3 day of heat. By this time the jack's sperm count is greatly reduced and the breeding may not take. 3. You of course cannot put young jennets - under the age of two years in with jacks, or jennets that are related to the jack. Inbreeding miniature donkeys should NEVER be an option! 4. Some jacks constantly harass, chase and bite jennets even when they are in foal. This constant harassment and stress can easily cause abortions. 5. Some adult jacks look upon weanling jacks (3-4 months of age) as threats and may seriously injure them. 6. You should NEVER leave a jack with a jennet when she is giving birth. We've had several stories of jacks killing newborns.

Hand Breeding: Hand breeding takes more effort on your part which basically is the only negative. Jacks have their own pastures and are kept alone in them. They may object at first, but quickly become accustomed to being alone. If you have more than one jennet, the other jennet will usually ride (mount) the jennet that is in heat or the jennet in heat will go to the jack's fence line and urinate or chomp their mouths. When a jennet comes in heat, breeders generally wait until the 3rd day of heat and take the jennet and put her in with the jack. (If the jack is a biter, ALWAYS put a muzzle on the jack.) Let the jack breed the jennet once or twice and then remove her and put her back in her own pasture. Do this on day 3 and day 5 of her heat cycle. If you are breeding a jennet that has a foal on her side, never put the foal in with the jack and jennet as it could easily get hurt during the breeding process. Since the breeding process doesn't take long, the foal is usually only without Mom for 20-30 minutes.

Take everything into consideration when deciding how you want to do things and use your best judgement.

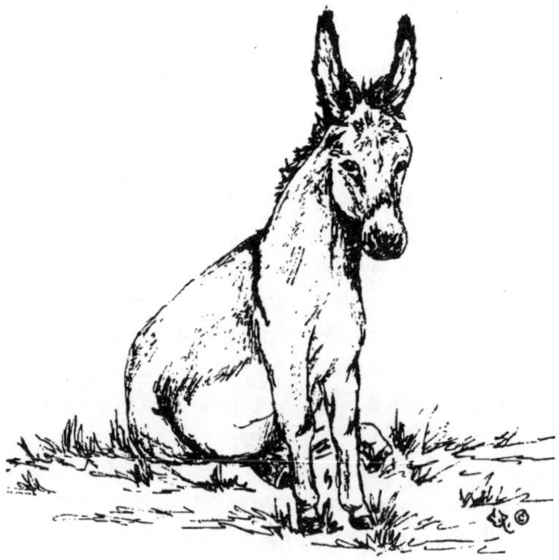

Chapter 2

The Pregnant Jennet

Breeding In "Foal Heat"

A jennet who has just foaled will come into heat about 9 days later, although this may range from about 6 to 18 days and is called "foal heat". Rebreeding at this time is very controversial but one which should have the pros and cons discussed.

The single most important factor that determines whether the jennet can be bred successfully during her foal heat is the condition of her reproductive tract after foaling. She should NOT be bred if she experienced a difficult foaling, retained the placenta for an extended period, or had any tearing, bruising or infection. If any of the above occurred, her reproductive tract may not be capable of supporting a new pregnancy. It should be noted that lacerations or tears to the vulva lips often occur in maiden jennets because of their failure to achieve sufficient relaxation.

Breeding a jennet who has just had her first foal, is not an acceptable practice. Most all are swollen and have a discharge. The discharge is not necessarily an infection, but a continuation of the cleansing and repair to the jennet's reproductive system. We have never been successful in getting a jennet rebred it she has a discharge.

It can be very difficult to determine when to breed in foal heat. Many jennets show signs of heat for two weeks so if you are hand breeding, you will not know when she is releasing an egg. Jennets who have had 3 or more foals, are fairly stretched, have no swelling or discharge, may be a candidate for breeding at this time. It should be noted that in a recent survey conducted by Miniature Donkey Talk Magazine, people stating they breed in foal heat, achieved an approximate 35% conception rate.

Getting The Story Straight on Pregnancy Testing

The primary reason for performing the pregnancy test is obviously to determine whether a donkey is pregnant. From a management standpoint, there are also several secondary reasons why pregnancy tests are helpful: #1 Pregnancy tests help prevent breeding during gestation - if the pregnant jennet shows *signs* of heat. #2 They increase the chances of getting a jennet settled before the season is over. #3 Pregnancy tests minimize the time an outside jennet must spend at the jack owner's farm.

There are several methods of detecting pregnancy and each varies with respect to cost, convenience, and accuracy. A very few pregnant jennets show signs of estrus throughout gestation, while some nonpregnant ones fail to show estrus due to a number of possible physiological and psychological problems. I have listed below several methods and tests for detecting pregnancy, in terms that we can all understand, as they refer to Miniature Donkeys.

Rectal Palpation: Rectal palpation is totally unacceptable for Miniature Donkeys because of their small size. It is very easy to rupture the rectum during palpation resulting in peritonitis and causing the animals death. ***Rectal palpation ranks number one in AVMA malpractice liability claims*** (and this is primary for large horses, which gives you an idea of just how dangerous this practice is.) Some veterinarians, unfamiliar with miniatures, will suggest that you go this route not realizing themselves the harm they cause. Do not put your miniature jennets through this painful and dangerous practice.

MIP-TEST (Mare Immunological Pregnancy Test): This used to be a widely used test on horses and some test kits are still on veterinarian shelves. The University of Pennsylvania - New Bolton Center states that this test does not work on donkeys as donkeys do not produce enough of the hormone "gonadotropin" to make the test viable.

Progesterone Test: This test is done to see how much progesterone is circulating in the blood. The level is very low when the jennet is in heat and a bit higher between heats. The test can be done 18 to 25 days after mating. If the progesterone is very low, it can be determined that she is not pregnant. If it is high, she *could* be pregnant, she *could* be in between heats, or she *could* be in a false pregnancy. This test is good for telling you that the jennet is NOT bred, but isn't specific for positive pregnancy.

PMSG TEST (Pregnant Mare Serum Gonadotrophin): This test is done between 50 and 80 days after conception. High levels of PMSG indicate that conception has occurred but do not necessarily mean that the jennet is still pregnant. Once the pregnant uterus starts making PMSG, and the jennet stayed pregnant for up to 5/6 weeks, she continues to produce PMSG even if the fetus is reabsorbed, dies, is aborted, or again if the jennet is experiencing a false pregnancy. As long as the uterus is making PMSG, she will not come back in heat so you will think she is pregnant.

**** Estrone Sulfate Test ****: I feel this is the test of choice especially for Miniature Donkeys. It is fairly new so your veterinarian may not be familiar with it. This test will not only detect pregnancy, but that the foal is alive and well. The test can be done anytime after 75 days FROM THE LAST

BREEDING DAY. The jennet's ovaries produce a small amount of ES even when she's not pregnant. The foal and placenta together make large amounts of the hormone. After 65 days, the levels rise dramatically and stay high throughout pregnancy. Because the foal itself produces the ES, it means that if the hormone level is high, the foal is alive. Jennets who abort or reabsorb the fetus show a rapid drop in ES concentrations. We at *Pheasant Meadow Farm* have had well over 100 of these tests done with 100% total accuracy.

Ultrasound: There are two methods to ultrasound an equine. The first is manually inserting the probe into the jennet's rectum in which the veterinarian guides the probe with her hand. Again, as with rectal palpation, this practice is unacceptable for miniatures. The second method involves shaving the belly area and ultrasounding through the stomach wall. It is recommended that Miniature Donkeys be ultrasounded after 55 days, however, a more experienced vet may be able to pick up a fetus much sooner. Although charges for this test vary greatly throughout the country, our personal vets charge us $40 per jennet.

Bet Labs Pregnancy Testing

Have your vet draw blood and send to: **BET Laboratories, 6174 Jacks Creek Road, Lexington, KY 40515 (606) 273-3036.**

BET explains Pregnancy Testing In The Mare

1. Progesterone assay alone will not confirm the mare is pregnant. Progesterone assays will tell you if the mare is producing enough of this hormone to maintain the pregnancy.

2. BET prefers to test for PMSG (pregnant mares serum gonadotropin) also known as Equine Chorionic Gonadotropin, when mares are between 45 and 90 days pregnant. This test has approximately a 5% false negative rate and 10% false positive rate. PMSG values above 1 I.U. per ml are considered positive, however, normal values are between 10 and 100 I. U. per ml. Mares which are below 10 I.U. but pregnant may be at risk of losing the pregnancy unless maintained on progestin therapy.

3. From 90 days to term, total estrogen assays are used to confirm pregnancy and monitor fetal viability. This test includes estrone sulfate and is approximately 99% accurate. Total estrogen assays work best between 100 days and two weeks prior to foaling.

Days of pregnancy	Total Estrogens Mean Concentrations (pg/ml)
barren/open	50-50
90-100	75
100-110	205
110-120	356
120-130	469
130-140	857
140-150	1040
150-320	greater than 1000

NOTE: Approximately two weeks before foaling, estrogen levels fall rapidly to approximately 300.00 pg/ml.

Rectal Palpation - Just Say NO!

*(Ed Note: Anyone who has received **MDT** for any length of time knows that I am totally against rectal palpation of Miniature Donkeys to determine pregnancy. This article was written for LARGE HORSE MARES. Some people have stated that they use a tiny female veterinarian to palpate their mini's therefore, it is justified. This thought provoking article provides information on why palpation of a mini, by any sized veterinarian is not rational.)*

Palpation is a veterinary procedure which, although not complex in nature, requires tact and judgement. Although proficiency does demand manual dexterity borne of practice and confidence, there seems to be no greater likelihood of an inexperienced veterinarian inducing rectal perforations than an "old hand". What the newcomer lacks in experience he makes up for in extra caution.

Almost every practicing equine veterinarian has had an experience where he has induced - probably through no fault of his own - at least a partial rectal tear. Given the high mortality rate associated with such injuries, the mere suspicion that a tear has occurred is cause for immediate concern. *Rectal tears rank as one of the leading sources of veterinary malpractice lawsuits, according to statistics maintained by the American Veterinary Medical Association.*

Is it the responsibility of the veterinarian to warn the owner and/or manager of the potential dangers involved each time a mare is examined? Is an annual review of the risks sufficient? Or is it a procedure so commonplace [in large horse mares] that the risk is understood and accepted by all parties?

Rectal palpation [on horse farms] is a procedure that is carried on routinely throughout the breeding industry, but it is not without serious risk. The inner layer of the equine rectum is very fragile and can be easily damaged. Veterinarians attempt to minimize the risk of internal injury by "nonaggressive" palpation. The examiner allows his arm to go limp or even removes it from the rectum in the face of expulsive efforts by the mare.

The mare who is mildly resistant may be distracted sufficiently by using a twitch. A local anesthetic in the lubricating gel effectively inhibits straining in most instances. In extreme cases, epidural anesthesia may be necessary to repress not only the sensation but also the ability to actively strain. However, the potential side effects - risk of infection, incoordination after use - limit its application. There are some mares in whom rectal palpation is simply not practical. The risk of injury is greater than the reward.

In the face of continued or excessive resistance, it is necessary for the examining veterinarian to acknowledge the presence of serious risk and re-evaluate the need for the examination. This is the juncture at which a "simple" veterinary procedure takes on managerial and legal implications.

Although veterinarians palpate with their fingers as close together as possible, avoiding the use of a single pointed finger, the fingertips may cause some tears. In other instances, a more explosive situation involving the examiner's hand or forearm may result from the straining rectal tissue. With some incomplete tears, the mucosa may be so friable that it just splits "at the seams" in a couple of spots.

A veterinarian's suspicions of a tear will be confirmed by the presence of blood on his sleeve. Once the veterinarian acknowledges the fact that damage has occurred, he will proceed to discover how serious the problem might be. A first step is to examine the rectum using a glass or plastic vaginal speculum or a fibre-optic endoscope. After your veterinarian determines the extent of the damage, then the two of you must decide what medical steps are going to be taken. If the mare has suffered a complete rectal tear outside the peritoneal space, she is more likely to develop a massive abscess than deadly peritonitis, although both situations are life-threatening. If the perforation occurs in front of the area to which the peritoneum connects, it may only be a matter of hours before the mare dies an acutely painful death. At this point, there is no alternative except surgery: going in through the belly, flushing out whatever fecal material may be present, repairing the wound and administering high doses of antibiotics.

Anytime there appears to be even a remote possibility of damage, the prudent veterinarian immediately informs his client, then takes aggressive steps to either repair the damage or make some decisions about what to do. Such action usually involves more than giving the mare injections of antibiotics and painkillers.

When a complete rectal tear extends into the peritoneum, swift aggressive treatment is imperative, or death will surely follow. No matter how alarming the prospects, the potential for disaster is too great to ignore.

Reference: by Bobbie Lieberman

An Explanation for Estrous Behavior in a Pregnant Mare

Pregnant mares don't usually exhibit estrous behavior (obvious interest in a nearby stallion and strong signs of receptivity), but sometimes they do. Such behavior has caused many an owner to wonder if the mare is pregnant after all. The peculiar situation has been reported on for some *50* years, but without any explanation for the behavior. Now a study from the University of Wisconsin offers a very convincing possibility

The first finding on which the hypothesis is based is that estrous behavior during pregnancy is more common in mares with a female fetus than in mares with a male fetus; all 12 mares in which such estrous behavior was observed actually had female foals. Now, it is known that a combination of low progesterone concentration and a source of estrogens may result in estrous behavior. The source of that estrogen supply may indeed be the fetus, and in fact the female fetus may produce larger quantities of estrogens than the male.

As additional support for the hypothesis comes from the fetus itself. It is definitely known that an equine fetus has estrogen producing capability from Day 12 and that this increases during Days 12-20. This corresponds with the period of pregnancy in which signs of estrus are most commonly observed. Horse owners may want to do a bit of amateur sex-predicting on their own, just watch out for estrous behavior in a mare known to be pregnant. Then, perhaps, take bets on the gender of the anticipated offspring.

MDT Ed Note: I discussed this several years ago in MDT as I observed the same thing. We kept track of seven jennets who showed signs of estrus even though they were pregnant. Six had jennet foals, one had a jack foal. Signs of estrus in these jennets never lasted more than 3 days.

Reference: Cornell University College of Veterinary Medicine

Reproductive Complications

Reproductive complications can fall into several categories: management problems, physical conditions, infections, hormonal abnormalities and miscellaneous causes.

There are continual advances in diagnostic procedures. The fiberoptic endoscope enables veterinarians to directly view the inside of a jennet's uterus. Uterine adhesions and cysts, ovarian tumors and other problems can be seen, biopsied and treated. The ultrasound machine can view the entire reproductive tract. If physical examination fails to disclose a problem, your vet will want to perform lab tests.

Uterine cytology means the study of cells. Your vet will swab the uterus to obtain sample cells which are then examined under a microscope. Unusually high white blood cells will indicate inflammation in the uterus as well as bacteria associated with infections. A cytology generally costs between $25 and $60. A culture and sensitivity test is usually done at the same time - $30 to $60. Uterine fluid is smeared on a bacterial growth plate in the lab and kept warm for up to 72 hours to allow any microorganisms to grow. The lab will then run a test to determine which antibiotic must be used against the infection. If these tests show positive, your vet may want to recommend a uterine biopsy - $30 to $50. This involves the removal and evaluation of a tiny piece of uterine lining, detecting scarring and glandular damage.

The Barren/Repeat Breeder Jennet

You've bred that jennet any number of times. Maybe if you breed her more often during her heat cycle or you aren't breeding her at the right time. You don't have winter foaling facilities, so the time is getting near that you will simply have to wait until next year.

You are starting to think that you have a problem here, but where should you begin? You first need a good set of record books and if not, a superb memory. Your veterinarian is going to want to know how often she has been bred, on what days of her heat cycle, if she has foaled before, and on and on. He's going to want to know questions only a set of records will answer. His questions will help him in determining where the problem could possibly be and where to begin. Your record books will help in alleviating a lot of investigative work, ultimately saving you time and money.

Farm Overview

- ❑ **Looking at all jennets, are your overall conception rates good?**
- ❑ **Is your overall conception rate fairly poor?**
- ❑ **Did the jack you used to breed this jennet settle other jennets that were bred to him?**
- ❑ **Did the jack you used to breed this jennet leave other jennets open this year?**
- ❑ **Has this particular jack always had a very poor conception rate?**
- ❑ **Have you noticed a change in the number of jennets this jack normally gets bred to what he has settled this year?**
- ❑ **Is this jennet showing peculiar sexual behavior compared to other jennets?**
- ❑ **Have you changed your normal breeding practices to something different than what you normally do?**

In many cases, a quick scan of the overall picture may answer a lot of questions.

#1 Stop breeding this jennet. If you are right and she does have a problem, continuing to breed her may add other problems.

#2 Compare this jennet to other jennets on your farm. Is her open status the *exception* or does this problem seem to be *going around.* If it is *going around*, it may not be this jennet but a farm management problem.

#3 What is this jennet's medical history? Is she an older jennet? In horses, reproductive problems seem to start up around the age of 12 however, in donkeys there are no statistics. Donkeys live considerably longer than horses, so the term "aged" may not apply to jennets until they are in their late teens. Multiple pregnancies do put wear and tear on the reproductive tract. Is this jennet overly fat or too thin? Has she been seriously ill recently?

#4 Evaluate her foaling history. Has this jennet foaled every year or does her past history indicate that she only conceives every other year. Is it typical for this jennet to have difficulty in getting settled? If she has a foal on her side, is she psychologically too "bound" to her foal and carries on when separated from it? Did her last foaling proceed smoothly or were there problems. Were you there when she foaled? If not, you wouldn't know how much difficulty she did or didn't have. Was the placenta retained for more than two hours?

#5 Evaluate her breeding history. Has this jennet always had difficulty in conceiving? If you have not owned this jennet very long, you may not know the answer to this. You may not have a problem, this may be more of rule of thumb for this particular jennet.

#6 Specifically evaluate her estrous cycles this year. The normal estrous cycle, including estrus and diestrus is an average 21 to 23 days for miniature jennets. A significant deviation from this average may spell trouble. Does she display typical behavior during estrus? Could she possibly be a "silent heat" jennet or does she act like she's in heat all the time?

Lactational Anestrus

Lactational anestrus is not uncommon in miniature jennets. As long as these jennets have a nursing foal at side, they simply do not cycle. The hormone prolactin, which stimulates milk production, inhibits a follicle-stimulating hormone, which is necessary for growth of follicles. Wean the foal, and everything comes back to normal.

Estrus / Diestrus Cycles

The reproductively active jennet's estrous cycle is on average 21 to 23 days long. It is made up of a 5 day estrus (in-heat cycle) and a 16 to 18 diestrus (out of heat cycle). The length of diestrus is the important piece of information that you need. Any inflammation in the jennet's uterus usually causes diestrus to be shortened, bringing the jennet back into heat sooner than expected.

Diestrus is maintained by progesterone secreted by the corpus luteum. Injectable prostaglandin can be given to the jennet to shorten her diestrus and bring her into heat. If no injections of prostaglandin were given, shortened diestrus most likely means the uterus is inflamed.

Another factor that can shorten diestrus is a deficiency of progesterone. Assays for progesterone concentrations in the blood, using very accurate test kits, can be run by your vet right on your farm. Some jennets need progesterone treatments to support a pregnancy.

Early Embryo Loss

The term Early Embryo Loss means the pregnancy was terminated usually within the first 40 days of gestation. The exact cause is difficult to determine. The equine's age can be a determining factor as jennets in their late teens have a slighter higher incidence of loss than younger animals. On the other hand, yearling jennets on up to two year olds have an even higher incidence of loss. This may be mother nature's way of preventing pregnancy in animals who cannot physically or mentally carry an embryo to full term.

A healthy inside layer of the uterus is crucial as this is where the embryo embeds as it starts to develop. Endometritis (inflammation or infection of the inside wall of the uterus) is a major reason for early embryo loss. The infection may kill the embryo outright or may cause decrease in progesterone, which is necessary for pregnancy. Progesterone is a hormone produced which quiets uterine muscle contractions. If the jennet conceives, her system will detect the baby and will continue to produce progesterone. Note: Once an equine aborts, the presence of a certain hormone can inhibit her ability to conceive again for up to four months. Ulcer-like structures, called endometrial cups, form in the uterus and begin manufacturing the hormone PMSG on about the 35th day of pregnancy, and continue to do so until about day 100. If an equine aborts any time after the 40th day, the cups continue to manufacture the hormone, which seems to make conception almost impossible until after the 100th day.

A healthy jennet has a much better chance of carrying the embryo through this first stage of gestation. Equines which are very thin, carry a greater percentage of loosing the embryo. During breeding, the jennet should be at her ideal weight or slightly heavier. Dietary deficiencies are passed on to the foal making them weaker, have lower resistance to infection and often have defects in conformation.

Stress is an important factor in pregnancy loss and studies are currently under way in equines to determine just how much stress is harmful. It is thought that stress lowers progesterone levels, leading to embryo death. Stress also lowers the animal's resistance to disease.

Your jack should be a consideration in early embryo loss as he can transmit an infection from one jennet to another. Failure to get your jennets bred, should include an examination of him and his semen.

If a specific cause can be found for early embryo loss, prevention and treatment can be set in motion. In the case of progesterone deficiency, this can be provided either by injection or oral form. In the case of infection, lab tests can be done to find the specific antibiotic that will combat that specific bacteria, and infused in the uterus.

In all cases, early embryo death should be investigated so that the cause can be eliminated. Sometimes no specific cause can be determined, in which case, the loss should be accepted and the jennet rebred.

Causes of Abortion

The term abortion refers to the expulsion of the embryo or fetus between day 30 and 300 of pregnancy. Equines are much more susceptible to abortion than most other domestic animals. In the cow, the membranes surrounding the calf actually grow deeply into receptor sites in the uterine lining. By contrast, the membranes surrounding the equine foal only grow slightly into the mare's uterine lining. This makes disruption of the attachment much more likely.

If the foal is delivered after a gestation of more than 300 days, it is designated as a stillborn, premature, or full term, depending on the circumstances of the delivery. Stillbirth, for example, is the expulsion of a dead fetus that has reached what would normally be considered a viable stage of development.

Hormone Imbalances, i.e. progesterone deficiencies can be an important cause of habitual abortion. This form of abortion usually occurs between the fourth and fifth months. Hormones must be produced by the body in the right sequence and amount in order to get and keep her pregnant. If anything goes wrong with this series of hormonal changes, the fetus will be aborted. Your vet may recommend progesterone injections to help maintain pregnancy.

Equine Viral Rhinopneumonitis is a highly contagious disease. The disease is seen in young donkeys as a respiratory disease then appears in older equine, often some months later, as the cause of abortions late in pregnancy although it can cause abortions as early as the fifth month. The jennet may show no signs of infection but the virus invades the placental membranes and attacks the fetus. The fetus is usually aborted in about 3-12 weeks when it is no longer able to function physiologically. Miniature Donkeys should be vaccinated with Equine Rhinopneumonitis Vaccine in their 5th, 7th, 9th and 11th months of pregnancy.

Bacterial Infections may cause the jennet to abort early in the pregnancy. Often no signs are noticed in connection with one of these early abortions. Bacteria such as Staph, Strep, and E. Coli are among those causing this type of problem.

Breeding the pregnant jennet can cause abortion in any month. Most jennets stop cycling once they have conceived but some continue to cycle for one, or rarely, two months afterwards. If the pregnant jennet is bred, the cervical seal that maintains uterine stability will be disrupted and abortion occurs.

Rectal palpation to determine pregnancy has been documented as causing abortion in Miniature Donkeys for a variety of reasons but mainly due to the pain and stress during the process.

Jennets carrying twins often abort after the 6th month of pregnancy, although there are a few documented cases of the delivery of twins. Twin abortion is often preceded by premature udder development and the jennet may drip or run milk beforehand. Apparently at around 6 months, the twins reach the limits of uterine stretch or capacity and abort for that reason.

Fescue toxicity is a more common reason for abortions in horse mares than it is in donkey jennets. Fescue toxicity is caused by an alkaloid present in the grass during the lush stages of growth during the spring and early summer. It is rare for fescue grass to cause abortion in Miniature Donkeys but I have heard of it causing placentas to become too thick for a foal to break through on their own. Fescue is seldom a problem on pastures that contain only a small percentage of fescue. The grass is less palatable than other grasses and equines usually refuse to eat it unless nothing else is available.

Immature jennets may abort simply due to the fact that they cannot produce enough hormones and nutrients to produce a viable foal.

Trauma such as a kick, can cause abortion. The fetus is surrounded and protected by a cushion of fluid, however, a severe kick that hits the fetus directly may cause abortion. The aborted fetus usually displays a distinctive bruise at the site of injury. Severe stress due to overwork, fright or severe illness can also be responsible for abortion especially during the late stages of pregnancy.

Signs of abortion may be minimal, especially in the first month or two. You may happen to find a small, slippery sac and see a slight bleeding or dark brown discharge from the vulva. If you are not in the right place at the right time, you might not see anything at all. I firmly believe that mother nature has a hand in some abortions to rid the body of a defective foal when no other causes can be found.

An aborted fetus is expelled wrapped in its membranes. If you wish to have it examined to try to determine the cause of abortion, be sure to save the membranes as well because they are often more informative than the fetus as to what caused the problem. If the jennet has aborted a fetus and the membranes have not followed, be certain to call your veterinarian.

Foal Development in Utero

How do foals develop? ***Conception to Delivery***

If you're planning to breed your jennet/mare this year, you'll probably do quite a bit of research. First you'll decide on the stud, then determine the best time for breeding. Once you've crossed the hurdle of getting your jennet/mare bred, you may be thinking of how to prepare for the foal's birth.

What happens in the eleven to twelve months between breeding and foaling? Will you simply turn your jennet/mare out to pasture, knowing that nature will take its course and a foal will appear on time? Have you ever wondered just how that small embryo develops into a fetus and finally emerges as a living, breathing entity?

Your jennet's environment has a critical influence on the development of her foal. Nutrition and exercise, stress, drugs, and many other factors can critically affect the foal's growth.

Foal development can be divided into trimesters, or thirds of gestation (pregnancy). Another way to think of development is in stages, from conception to embryonic development and finally fetal growth.

CONCEPTION

The act of conception requires precise coordination and timing. During each heat cycle, the jennet's ovaries release one or more eggs into the ovarian tube (oviduct). Studies show that a double ovulation occurs from 15 to 30% of the time. After ovulation, the egg remains high in the oviduct, awaiting the arrival of a sperm cell.

During breeding, the stallion ejaculates directly into the jennet's uterus. Millions of tiny sperm begin their attempts at finding the egg. The sperm remain alive for up to two days. This is the reason behind the recommendation of breeding jennets/mares every other day during their heat cycle.

When a sperm cell penetrates the egg, the genetic material of stallion and jennet are blended to create a new individual. This primitive cell begins to divide even while it travels down the oviduct towards the body of the uterus.
About five or six days later, the fertilized egg enters the jennet's uterus. Rapid cell division continues as it floats freely there, moving from one horn (side) to the other at will.

THE EMBRYO

The embryo stage begins at about day 15 and continues through the end of the second month of pregnancy. This is a time of specialized changes, when the foal's different body systems are formed. By 30 days, the eyes, mouth, and most of the foal's body organs have begun to form. The tiny embryo is already recognizable as a donkey or horse about 40 days after conception.

While the foal's sex was determined at the time that the sperm and egg met, the sex organs don't begin to differentiate until 40 days of pregnancy. Between 50 and 70 days, it's possible to determine the sex of the fetus by careful ultrasonic examination.

The embryo must "eat" and eliminate wastes while it grows. This transfer occurs through the complex system of membranes which make up the placenta. As the embryo grows, it surrounds itself with a double-layered, sac-like structure. The inner amnion contains the foal, while the outer chorioallantois begins to attach to the uterus, forming the placenta. The result is that six tissue layers separate the jennet and fetus. Because of a specialized transport system, only particular substances are allowed to travel from the jennet's circulation to that of her unborn foal.

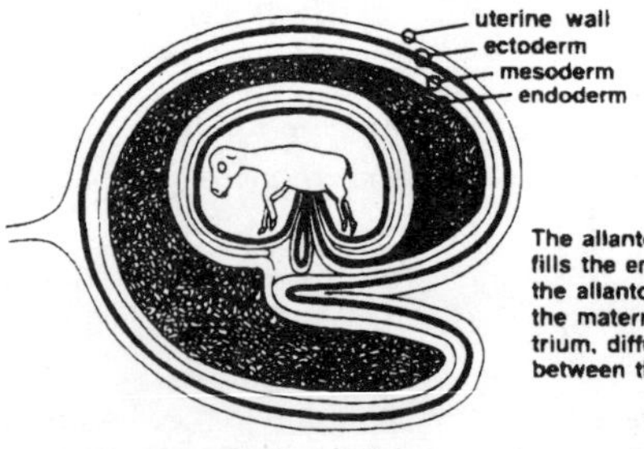

The allantoic cavity gradually fills the entire uterus. Where the allantochorion contacts the maternal uterine endometrium, diffuse attachment forms between the two tissues.

Many drugs can cross the placental barrier and affect the foal. Red blood cells from the jennet/mare deliver oxygen for transport to the fetus, but do not cross the placenta. Proteins such as disease-fighting antibodies are too large to cross the barrier. Instead, foals must receive their antibodies from colostrum, the jennet's first milk.

The tiny embryo is attached to the placenta only by the umbilical cord, so it can move about freely. Nutrients and oxygen are transferred to the fetus through the umbilical vein. The umbilical cord also contains the urachus. This tube drains urine out of the foal's bladder and into the area between the amnion and chorioallantois.

During the embryo stage, the developing foal is most susceptible to outside influences. As veterinarians are becoming better at diagnosing early pregnancy, it's become apparent that early pregnancy loss in the mare is a problem.

THREATS TO PREGNANCY

Before the use of ultrasound, pregnancy wasn't even diagnosed until at least four weeks along, the time when changes in the uterus, in the horse, can be felt with a rectal examination. Now the embryonic vesicle can be visualized as early as 10 to 14 days after breeding. Sequential ultrasonic examinations show us that at least 10% of all pregnancies are lost in the first eight weeks after conception.

Jennets that are very young or very old have a much greater risk of pregnancy loss. Uterine infections are another common cause of embryonic death.

Poor nutrition or undue stress placed on the jennet can lead to problems in the fetus. Illness or administration of certain drugs to the jennet can also harm fetal development.

All medications approved for use in equine will carry a statement on their labels concerning the drug's use in pregnant mares. If you aren't sure, don't use the product! Extensive studies have not yet been performed in horses, but drugs that can be harmful to embryonic development in other species include hormones, excessive vitamins, phenylbutazone, and several antibiotics.

On the other hand, many well-intentioned owners neglect routine care for fear of harming the unborn fetus. Regular deworming and vaccination is essential for the health of both jennet and foal! Ask your veterinarian to outline a program for your pregnant jennet.

Twin conceptions are frequently lost. Even though there are a high percentage of double fertilizations, we don't see many twin foals born. The jennet's uterus is usually capable of nurturing only one fetus all the way to term.

Nature frequently takes care of the twin problem. One study showed that in 85% of twin conceptions, one of the pair was lost before 50 days along, leaving the other to develop normally. Twins that survive longer than this are usually aborted later or are stillborn.

GROWTH

Day 60 through delivery is considered the fetal growth period. The lips and feet become recognizable by two months; at three months, hooves have developed. The tiniest hairs begin to form during the sixth month, and fine hair covers the foal's body at nine months.

A recent study showed that the fetus is much more active than anyone had thought. At 60 days, mouth, head and limb movements occur regularly. The 70- to 80-day-old fetus is extremely active, swimming about with an occasional somersault.

While the fetus lives in the womb, its circulatory system is adapted to receiving oxygen from the placenta. During the last months of gestation, the fetal lungs begin to mature, preparing for the sudden change to breathing.

Up until about five months of pregnancy, the jennet requires only a good-quality diet at the same level that a non-pregnant jennet would receive. Very little additional nutrition is required, and extra calories will only add extra weight.

The greatest increase in fetal size -- about 65% of its growth --occurs during the last three months of gestation. This is the time period when the jennet's nutrition level should be analyzed carefully and increased <u>only</u> if there is a need.

FEEDING THE UNBORN FOAL

Calcium and phosphorus requirements increase, and the jennet/mare's caloric intake rises 12 to 15%. Each individual will have slightly different energy (calorie) requirements; use the jennet's body condition as your guide.

Recent studies have focused on the effects of the jennet's nutrient intake on the foal's nutritional status at birth. Some vitamins and minerals are not available in the jennet's milk in adequate quantities for the foal. Until creep feeding begins, the foal relies on body stores of certain nutrients which were collected during its time in the womb.

One researcher found that mineral deposits in the foal's body were greatest during the 10th month of pregnancy. During the 11th month, protein deposition was highest, and almost 50% of the iron was deposited.

At birth, most of this iron is in the foal's blood. This means that blood loss at birth (as when the umbilical cord is prematurely cut or torn) could lead to a deficiency in iron.

An excess of certain vitamins and minerals can be just as harmful as any deficiency. For example, too much vitamin A and D can interfere with the jennet/mare's utilization of calcium and phosphorus; copper, magnesium and zinc all must be balanced in order for each mineral to perform its function.

A jennet that is receiving a good plane of nutrition will probably take in plenty of vitamins and minerals for the foal's use. Precise nutritional guidelines have been drawn up by the National Research Council; ask your veterinarian for advice.

ULTRASOUND

Ultrasound has many uses in an equine breeding program. The ultrasonic image is formed by way of sound waves which are emitted from a transducer and bounce back at different speeds depending on the density of the object. Pregnancy in the jennet can be detected by ultrasound as early as ten to fourteen days, when the embryonic vesicle (sac) is first apparent. The size of the embryo is evaluated over time to be sure that it is developing normally.

The embryo within the vesicle is first seen after 20 days. Fetal heartbeats are readily discernible as early as 22-24 days of pregnancy. The sex of a fetus can also be determined with an ultrasound exam. The fetal genitals are visible and can be differentiated at about day 60 of pregnancy.

Recently, ultrasound-guided amniocentesis has been attempted on mares. Analysis of the fluid surrounding the fetus yields valuable information about its health and well-being. Amniocentesis has been an essential part of human prenatal testing for some time. Much research remains to be done before this technique can be adapted for practical use in the mare.

DELIVERY TIME

How do the jennet and foal "know" when the time is right for birth? A complex system of hormonal changes and chemical interactions between the jennet and foal begin the preparation for birth.

The fetus signals that it's ready for birth by releasing corticosteroid hormones. Other hormones in the jennet undergo drastic changes at the same time.

The result is that the udder fills with colostrum; the vulva relaxes and swells, so that it is capable of stretching to accommodate delivery of the foal; and finally the cervix dilates.

The jennet "breaks water" when the allantois ruptures, releasing lubricating fluid to ease delivery of the foal. The whitish sac containing the foal, which first appears at the vulva, is the amnion. If the red chorioallantois appears first, it means that the placenta has prematurely separated from the uterus -- an emergency, since the foal no longer is receiving its oxygen supply.

At birth, the foal's body goes through dramatic changes. The force of delivery pushes fluid out of the foal's lungs. The first breath requires extreme force, since all the airways are collapsed and wet. While the fetus was in the womb, its blood took up oxygen from the placenta. Now, suddenly, blood must travel through the foal's lungs to gather up life-giving oxygen. This is accomplished by dramatic changes in blood flow. Certain vessels and openings between them close down, having done their job for months but now becoming useless.

Transfer of blood from the placenta through the umbilical cord to the fetus continues for some time after actual delivery. A large percentage of the foal's blood supply can be lost if the cord is broken prematurely.

After birth, the umbilical vessels dry up and the urachus closes down. Contamination of the umbilical vessels before they close can lead to severe infection in the foal; this is prevented by application of iodine to the navel. Failure of the urachus to close, or patent urachus, leads to urine dripping out of the navel; sometimes surgical correction is required.

The placenta, or afterbirth, is passed within a few hours. You may notice a brownish rubbery structure, the hippomane, lying with the placenta. Hippomanes are believed to be formed from deposits of minerals and proteins. The Greek translation of this word is "horse madness," and the hippomane itself has an uncertain function.

Reference: By Carin Smith, DVM Green Grass Syndicated Features

The Hormones of Pregnancy

From conception until about day 150, the mare's ovaries produce the hormone progesterone, which helps the body to maintain pregnancy. This function is slowly taken over by the placenta, which begins to produce progesterone from day 60 onwards. Levels of this hormone rise gradually during pregnancy, and fall dramatically at birth. Progesterone levels can be used to diagnose pregnancy.

Pregnant mare serum gonadotropin (PMSG) is another important hormone produced during pregnancy. Special cells from the fetus attach to the placenta in circular areas that are called endometrial cups. The cups, which release PMSG, begin to form at around day 40 and persist until 100 days of pregnancy. Measurement of PMSG in the mare's blood is the basis for one popular pregnancy test.

Estrogen levels in the mare begin to rise around the third month of pregnancy, then fall just before birth. Estrogens can be measured in the mare's milk, urine, blood, and even manure, providing another possibility for a pregnancy test.

Prostaglandin levels rise sharply just prior to the beginning of labor. This hormone works with oxytocin to help expel the foal at birth.

Oxytocin is also released during the birth process. This hormone is used by veterinarians to help induce delivery in some mares or to stimulate uterine contractions in mares with retained placentas. Oxytocin stimulates milk let-down as well.

INFECTION

One of the first things your vet will look for is discharge from the vulva which can suggest infection. An infection can still be present without a discharge. If there is a discharge, the vet will want to determine what type of discharge it is. The vet will look closely at the vulva and its muscle tone. If the vulva fails to form a complete seal, it could allow foreign matter to enter, contaminating the vagina. The bodies natural defenses begin to fight off this bacteria and will also look on sperm as bacteria and will kill it off.

Sometimes doing a **uterine culture** to determine the type of bacteria can be frustrating. Some types of bacteria are very difficult to grow in labs. However, at the present time there are no alternatives available.

Jennets with **excessive progesterone** in the systems may have normal ovarian activity but the excess hormone may be just enough to keep the cervix too tight, preventing semen from getting into the uterus after breeding. On the other hand, if the cervix is too tight as a result of scar tissue, this could spell disaster when a full term foal tries to come through the narrowed cervix.

An ultrasound is a good way to look for cysts and screening the uterus for fluid. Since most bacteria that infect the uterus are to some degree, pus producers, and since infection is usually irritating and inflammatory, a quick ultrasound can confirm your vet's suspicions.

Another way to determine valuable information is **cytology**, where the vet prepares a microscope slide from a swab of the vagina, cervix or uterus. The examination under a microscope can reveal inflammation, mucus, pus, bacteria and various other clues to determine the health of the reproductive tract.

Reference: Dr. Carin Smith, Author of EASY HEALTH CARE FOR YOUR HORSE.

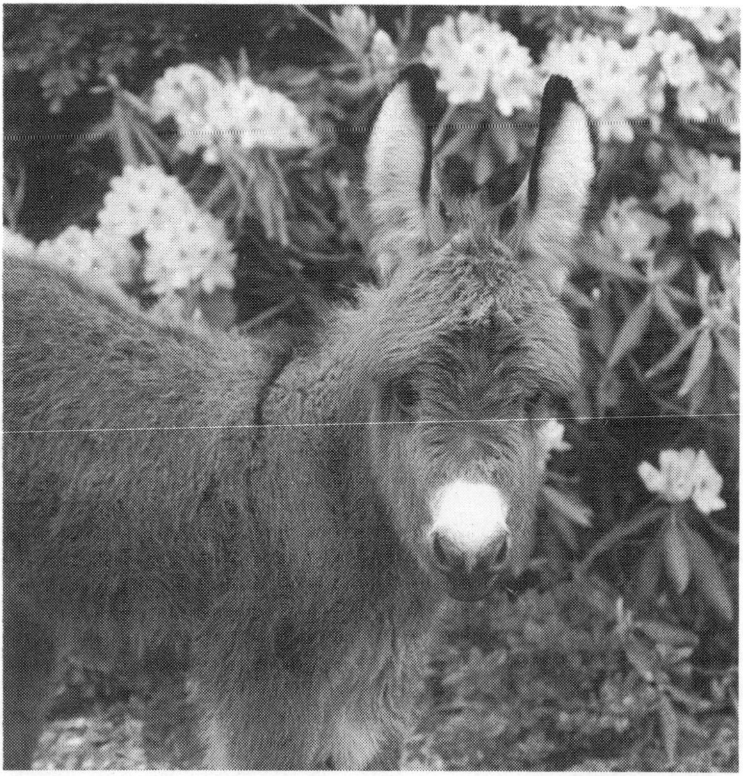

Winter Care of the Pregnant Jennet

Contrary to popular belief, feeding grain will not appreciably increase a donkey's body warmth, but feeding increased roughage (hay) will. The heat of digestion (in terms of calories) is greater and lasts longer from hay than from concentrates. It is the fermenting hay inside the belly that creates heat. It is most beneficial to feed a donkey several hours in advance of a winter storm rather than during it. Immediately after a large meal, blood is concentrated around and in the digestive tract, rather than in the muscles where it is needed for warmth. DO NOT drastically increase a pregnant jennet's feed, just because she is pregnant. She should maintain the weight level (unless she was underweight) at the time she was bred. Jennet's basic nutritional needs do not increase until the last 3 months of pregnancy but even then her feed should not be increased unless you notice her losing weight.

- ❑ DO feed good quality grain if feeding poor quality hay
- ❑ DO keep hooves trimmed as excess weight is hard on limbs
- ❑ DO keep up with regular vaccination schedules
- ❑ DO keep up with normal worming routine, however do not worm more often than every two months and not during her six weeks of pregnancy
- ❑ DO keep an unfrozen supply of fresh water available

- ❑ DON'T feed the jennet for two just because she is in foal
- ❑ DON'T let out on icy ground where she could slip and fall
- ❑ DON'T keep in very close knit quarters with other donkeys where she could get kicked, however, do not separate her from any buddies.
- ❑ DON'T feed wet or moldy hay
- ❑ DON'T groom excessively - dirt is a natural weatherproofing
- ❑ DON'T stall in an air-tight barn as lack of ventilation can cause respiratory problems.

Hypothyroidism
misdiagnosed and misunderstood

Hypothyroidism -- insufficient levels of thyroid hormones -- is difficult to diagnose. The accuracy of tests for the problem is questionable, and there are questionable effects of treatment when the ailment is misdiagnosed.

Thyroid hormones control protein synthesis. They are responsible for the overall metabolism of the animal and have bearing on the animal's energy level. Hypothyroidism is due either to insufficient levels of thyroid hormones or inappropriate release of hormones from the thyroid gland.

Signs of hypothyroidism include lethargy, muscular weakness, decreased exercise tolerance and goiter. Obesity, cresty neck, frequent bouts of laminitis, poor hair coat, mare infertility and foal tendon problems have all been reported to be associated with hypothyroidism, but are not scientifically documented.

Although the frequency of hypothyroidism is unknown, many horses and donkeys are placed on treatment -- which consists of thyroid hormones given as a feed additive -- for lack of other diagnosis. Symptoms often remain unexplained, and hypothyroidism can't be ruled out.

The test for hypothyroidism adds to the confusion. The easiest laboratory test measures T4, or sometimes T3 thyroid hormone levels in a single blood sample. There are many variables in using this method of testing.

For one, some forms of hormones are active, others are inactive, yet both affect the test. Some commonly used drugs, such as bute, and some diets have been reported to cause low levels of thyroid hormones. Thus the tests do not give an exact quantity of the active form and often are inaccurate.

To add to the confusion, there exists a multi-tiered feedback mechanism in the body for regulating the amount of hormones released by the thyroid gland.

There are natural daily and monthly fluctuations of the forms of hormones in the body. A single low-serum level of T4 or T3 does not prove that the animal is suffering from hypothyroidism.

The best means of measuring the function of the thyroid balance in the equine is to take repeated blood samples over a period of time. This helps to avoid gauging therapy on a singular low or high level that may only reflect a normal variation in an otherwise normally functioning thyroid gland.

Testing is also done by stimulating the thyroid to release thyroid hormones by giving a thyroid stimulating hormone (TSH).

TSH is normally produced by the pituitary gland in the course of a cascade of events that cause the thyroid gland to release hormones. Determining if the gland responds with an appropriate increase is accomplished by monitoring hormone levels in the blood after TSH is administered. Though this test is unquestionably more accurate, the TSH is only available for clinical use.

Supplementing horses and donkeys with a synthetic thyroid hormone works, but, in fact, it could lead to more problems than it solves.

Excessive supplementation can lead to decreased production of natural thyroid hormones. Normal mechanisms that detect the supplemental hormones conclude that it's naturally produced and may suppress the activity of the thyroid gland.

Supplementation may actually cause hypothyroidism, with the animal's body adjusting to and becoming dependent on the outside source of thyroid hormones. Other researchers, however, feel the synthetic thyroid supplement used in equine is not detected by the body and there is no risk associated with supplementation.

Excessive supplementation in humans causes heart palpitations and other cardiac effects associated with changes in the cardiac muscle. Whether such effects occur in the equine is unknown.

There simply is not enough known about the function and regulation of thyroid hormones in the horse to consider hypothyroidism as a common condition or one to treat with "best guess" supplements.

Until more research is done and better testing developed, diagnoses should only be based on a combination of laboratory values, physical signs and response to therapy, keeping the risks of that therapy in mind.

Reference: Written by Mike Beyer, D.V.M.

The Older Jennet

With each passing pregnancy the older jennet's reproductive tract goes through more wear and tear. Most of us know that there are many many miniature jennets still producing foals well into 20 years of age. Some of these jennets have only had three or four foals and others have delivered foals yearly since they were three years old. The jennet who has delivered year after year tends to eventually lose muscle tone, develop cysts and scar tissue.

Cysts can cause problems when they grow large enough or numerous enough to take up significant space in the uterus. They can obstruct the passage of a tiny embryo as it attempts to move throughout the uterus.

Scar tissue gradually replaces the rich glandular tissue that usually supports the growing placenta. The more scar tissue present, the less completely and securely the placenta can attach. There are basically no known cures for scar tissue.

The loss of muscle tone within the uterus can prevent a jennet from hanging onto an embryo. Some say that giving the jennet a year off from foaling may help but the very state of pregnancy tends to keep the uterine immune system sharp. A year off, and an older jennet may end up with a severely infected uterus.

Chapter 3

Getting Ready For The Foal

Foaling Kit Checklist

Your foaling stall should be equipped with soft rubber feed and water **buckets**. The soft rubber will absorb the impact of an unsteady or playful foal. Water buckets should be hung high enough off the ground where a foal cannot stick its head into it. Feed buckets should be removed after the jennet has eaten. Make sure your stall does not contain hazards which can trap a tiny hoof. One often unnoticed area is the space below your stall door. If there is a gap there, nail on a temporary board.

You can most likely expect your foal to arrive at night so you should have some lighting in your stall. The **lightbulb** should not be so bright that it hurts the newborn's eyes. You should have a bright bulb on hand for use in the case of emergency.

In winter and early spring, you will want to add two to four **heat lamps** to the stall. These are to be hung from the ceiling at a distance of 5 feet above the stall bedding (not the dirt floor).

For the actual birth, you will need a **flashlight**, bottle of **iodine**, **water soluble lubricant and sterile rubber gloves** (in case you have to enter your hand in the birth canal to help pull), **equine thermometer**, **terry cloth towels**, and a **shot glass** to apply iodine to the newborn's navel cord.

First time mothers at times can be difficult to deal with so you should have a suitable **halter and lead rope** on hand.

You will need a **shovel** to remove the placenta once the mother passes it. The placenta should be placed in a bucket and saved for at least 24 hours in case your vet wants to examine it. If the mother develops complications after the birth, the placenta is the first thing your vet will want to see.

A **baby bottle** should be on hand in case the foal cannot quite get the hang of nursing or the mother rejects her foal and will not let it nurse. In either case, you must milk the mother and feed the foal yourself. A **lambs nipple** works much better than a human baby nipple or equine nipple.

Have a **foal blanket** on hand. It may be needed to help a weak foal get through a stressful birth or during cold weather for the first few weeks. If you do not have a miniature foal blanket (horse foal blankets are too big) you may use a dog sweater - size 22 for newborns, size 24 for two week olds. Buy the economy priced ones that do not have the neck set in separately as it will need to be able to stretch a lot in the neck area to get it on. You can also buy dog coats that have a strap under the belly and around the back. Make sure the strap fits snug so that the foal cannot get a hoof caught up in it.

Be prepared! The foaling process is a wonderful and exciting time and not the time to be upset with yourself for not having these items available.

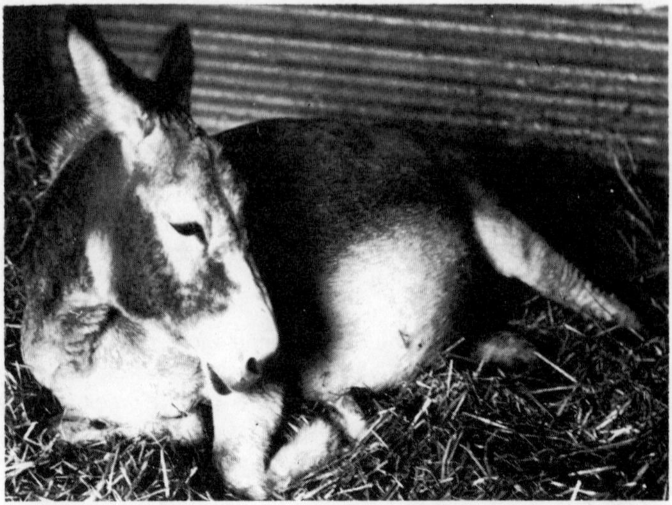

"...just hang in there until they go back to the house..."

When *Will* That Foal Arrive?

I'm sure many of you, as I, have spent weeks on end and many sleepless nights waiting for that jennet to foal. With the use of some very simple tools an owner can now somewhat predict when foaling time is near. Experienced breeders can usually tell delivery will take place within 48 hours by the fullness of the jennet's teats. This however, takes experience which new owners do not have. Also if you are a new owner and must go out of town for a day or two, the test below can help relieve your mind that your jennet has a few more days to go.

With a few water hardness test strips and a little of the jennet's milk, the approximate number of days left in the pregnancy can be predicted.

A study was done by Texas A & M University during their 1986 foaling season. As the animal approaches the birth, the calcium ion concentration in her milk will increase. With the use of the water hardness test strips the level of calcium concentration in the milk can be determined. The test strips have four color zones which will change from green to red-violet as the calcium increases. The more zones that change color, the closer the jennet is to foaling.

You should not be concerned about stealing the jennet's precious colostrum from the foal. Jennets produce much more than adequate amounts for the foal at birth. You will only milk a very small amount from the jennet. The test is called **Predict-A-Foal** and is manufactured by Animal Healthcare Products companies where you purchase your vaccines and sells for about $30.00. They only include 15 test strips for 15 tests. We cut the strips - lengthwise - in half which will give you 30 tests. You can order more test strips from EM Science, 111 Woodcrest Road, Cherry Hill, N.Y. 08034.

We have performed this test on numerous jennets to test for accuracy. At best, the test is excellent in telling you that you will not have a foal within a week but also that you will probably have a foal within a week. For those of you totally confused, if only one or two of the blocks on the strip changes color, you will in all probability not have a foal within 7 days. If all the blocks on the strip change color, you will most likely have a foal during the next 7 days.

How Close to Foaling Is She?

I get many calls asking of telltale signs of impending foaling. Some of you call me after three or four weeks telling me that your jennet FINALLY foaled! This is way too many sleepless nights!

There are several warning signs, however, I can assure you that not all jennets follow the rule books. Horse mares usually only have a two week leeway in gestation. Donkey jennets can carry a foal which can be termed "normal gestation" from 11-1/2 months to 13 months.

The most important thing I tell people is that you must KNOW your jennet. Know her idiosyncrasies, her eating habits and her social habits. This will tell you a lot. You must observe your jennet on a daily basis for an appropriate amount of time. You will then be able to notice telltale behavior changes. We always keep notes on these behavior changes and find that jennets will normally act the same way year after year.

I find that most jennets eat right up until maybe an hour before foaling. They will then do a lot of walking around, smelling the ground, and generally act like they're looking for that perfect spot to lay down. Maiden jennets are more apt to stop eating two to four hours before foaling simply because they are having such dramatic hormonal changes occurring and simply do not understand why they feel the way they do.

Warning: *Any jennet can foal without any sign; Any jennet can deliver without "waxing up"; Any jennet can foal with a small milk bag.*

During the last few weeks you will notice the muscles on either side of the tail will slacken. This allows the pelvic bones to move in preparation for foaling.

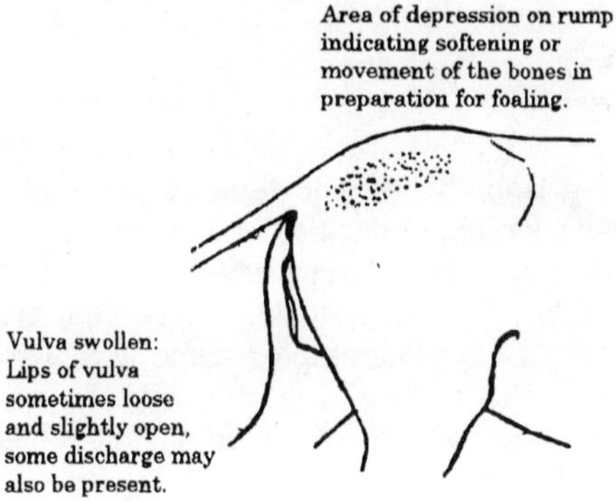

During the last two weeks (in some cases only the last day or two) in particular, your jennet will stand off to herself. Any other jennet approaching her will get a "look that could kill" with ears laid flat back. Fortunately she will not act this way with her human owners.

I have learned to heavily rely on the jennet's bag and teats. I would say 90% of the time we here at *Pheasant Meadow Farm* can predict foaling within 2 days from changes in the jennet's bag and teats. Jennets will usually start to bag up six to seven weeks before foaling. Many of them will have a half a bag on them and then all of a sudden completely lose it for three or four days, then bag up again over night. To notice changes in the bag, you must feel and observe your jennet's bag at least twice a day. *Important Note:* We have found that feeling a maiden (never foaled before) jennet's milk bag is very helpful when her foal goes to nurse the first time. Many maiden jennets object to being touched there and is one reason they will reject a foal. They do not understand what the foal is trying to do. After several weeks of you ever so lightly, touching her bag, she will become accustomed to it and will be less lightly to reject a foal.

Many jennets "wax up" from three days to several hours before foaling. This term actually refers to dry milk on the end of the teat. This is not a reliable sign as I have had jennets do this three and four weeks before foaling. This waxing up is natures way of stopping colostrum from dripping out of the teat. Most people who have never had a foal before do not realize just how full and hard a jennet's bag can become just prior to foaling. She will object to you touching her there after a while because it is so swollen and sore. Within three days of foaling, the teats will also fill with milk and become elongated. Before this happens and during your routine check of this area, you will be able to run your fingers across her teats with ease. When they become filled with milk, you will no longer be able to do this. Many jennets will have a very hard bag in the morning and then after walking around during the day, will have considerably less of a bag at night. The day that her bag is just as full at night, is when you should be on red alert.

Below are photos of a jennet's bag and teats to show you the extreme change that takes place just prior to foaling. I think this will help many first time owners to better know when exactly their jennet is going to foal. (I would like to thank "Chi Chi" for exposing herself for this photos.) I particularly picked Chi Chi to photograph as she was a maiden jennet. Maiden jennets have smaller bags and teats and although the change is more evident in jennets who have foaled before, I thought this was a better case study for you to observe.

Another word of warning. Donkeys are well known to be able to stop their first stage of labor because of human interference. We watched a jennet on our barn to house TV monitors go into her first stage of labor. We went down to the barn and very quietly stood inside the stall and simply watched as the front hooves of the foal appeared. She continued to lay down however, all contractions stopped. After 15 minutes, we left and went back to the house to watch her on the monitor. Within two minutes of our departure, she continued with her contractions and had a normal delivery.

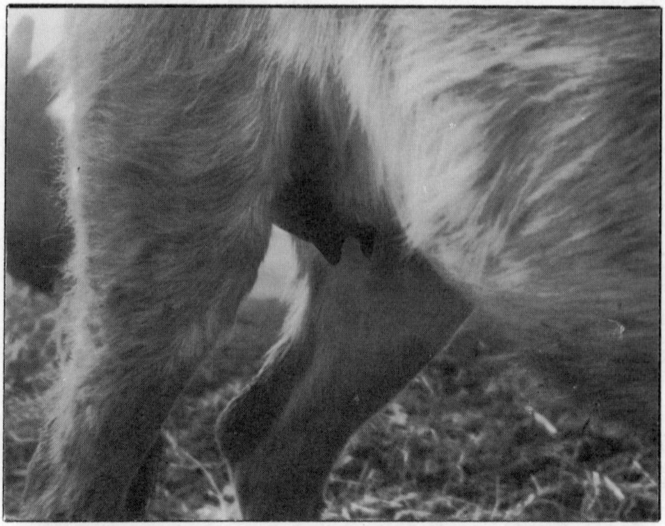

Jennet's bag and teats 3 weeks before foaling

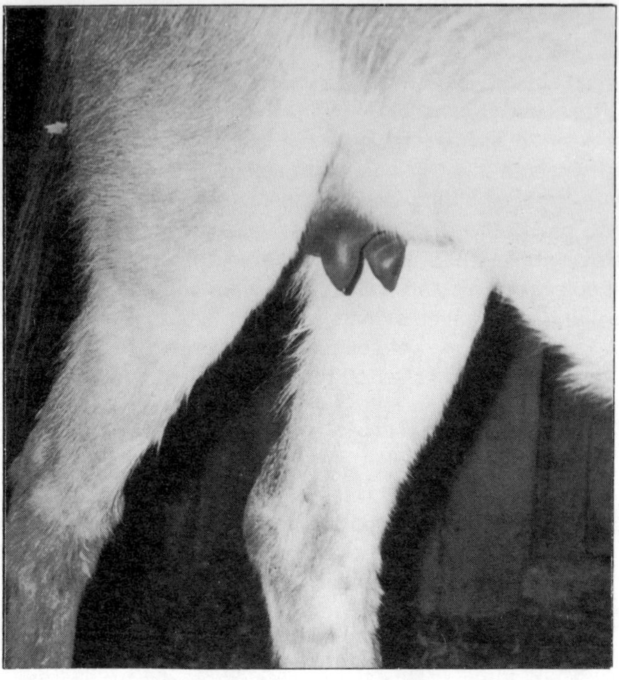

Top: Jennet's bag and teats 3 weeks before foaling Bottom: Photo showing fullness of jennets teats, six hours before foaling

The time frame just before your jennet foals is about as nerve-wracking as it gets. We get many phone calls asking exactly what indicates if the jennet will foal that day. Get real! If I knew that, I'd have a lot less (dyed) gray hairs from lack of sleep! I am to the point now, where I can tell 90% of the time if I'm going to have a baby born within 48 hours. That takes LOTS of experience and you must know your jennet and her personality *very well* to notice the sometimes suddle changes. Milk bags and teats are still good indicators.

Regarding the jennet:

1. Check with your vet regarding diet during the last months of pregnancy. He can evaluate your feeding program and also the weight and health status of your jennet. Does your jennet need to be on grain with selenium added? Are other minerals deficient in your area that should be added to her diet?

2. Your jennet should have been on a Rhino vaccination program to help prevent abortion. These vaccinations need to be given in the 5th, 7th, 9th, and 11th month.

3. Your jennet also should have a tetanus and 4-way vaccination booster approximately 6 weeks before foaling.

Regarding the stall:

1. You should have a very clean stall available - no smaller than 8' by 10'. Previous dirty bedding should be removed and the flooring covered with clean, dust-free straw. Do not use wood shavings. Shavings stick to a wet newborn foal. During warm spring or summer days, if your jennet goes in to labor during daylight, there is nothing wrong with her foaling outside preferably in a clean grassy area and obviously where no other animals can bother her. It's much better in appropriate weather, that a jennet foal outside on a clean pasture (in a spot she can get away from other donkeys and other animals) than in a stall.

2. Review every inch of your stall as it pertains to foal safety. Is the door of your stall a few inches off the ground - just enough to catch a tiny leg or hoof in? If so, nail a temporary board to it. Look for protruding nails. Newborns make numerous attempts to stand up after they are born and many times fall against walls. Attached the water bucket at least a foot off the ground. You wouldn't want your foal to fall head first into the bucket. Do your stall walls have boards with gaps in between that could also entrap a tiny hoof? If so, nail plywood around the sides of the stall. Never hang a hay net in a foaling stall. If you do not have a metal hay rack, put hay on the floor.

3. When you think your foaling stall is in good condition, sit on the floor and look for drafts or the smell of ammonia - both dangerous for a newborn. If the weather is cold, you should have several heat lamps hung up. Hang heat lamps a minimum of 5 feet above the bedding.

4. If you do not have a stall monitoring system, put a night light in the stall and arrange for a peep hole from outside the stall. When you go down to check on your jennet, you will not have to turn bright lights on and open loud doors. The reason most animals foal at night is because they are waiting to be alone and undisturbed!

Regarding your medical kit:

1. You should have at least two clean towels on hand. If the birth occurs in cold weather you may want to quickly towel dry the foal. (The key word here is "quickly".) Also have on hand your iodine to dip the navel. Putting a little iodine in a shot glass and holding it up against the foal's navel works well.

Regarding the next day:

A lot depends on the weather. I like to keep a jennet and her newborn stalled for at least the first 12 hours. They get to know each other and bonding between mother and baby takes place. After 12 hours, and weather permitting, I like to get the foal outside. I want that baby doing some running and jumping to get any remaining fluid out of their lungs. If the weather is cold, I'll put a foal blanket on the baby. (I never let foals get wet until they are 2 weeks old. Their coats are like cotton and absorb water and can take up to 12 hours to dry.) If the weather is bad, either very cold or very hot or flies are bothering the baby, I may let them in and out of their stall five times a day. We let the mothers and their newborns out in our foaling pasture which contains expectant mothers and mothers with foals on their side. New mothers are extremely protective and will keep other foals and adults away from their newborns. We always stall the mother and her newborn at night for at least the first two weeks. The mother and baby are secure and can get a good nights sleep and do not need to worry about other donkeys or animals during the night.

Be prepared for your new foal and you'll find that you will enjoy the experience much more.

Countdown to Foaling

<u>30 DAYS BEFORE</u>

Your jennet should be at her intended foaling location four to six weeks before her due date. She will be exposed to foreign organisms and will develop antibodies to these new bacteria and viruses, passing them along in her colostrum to her newborn.

Also now is the time to administer all vaccinations (Tetanus, Flu, Rhino and Equine Encephalomyelitis). This will provide high levels of protection for her at foaling and for the baby in its first several months of life. Equine Rhino vaccine used to reduce incidence of abortion will provide protective respiratory antibodies in the colostrum. Deworm your donkey SIX WEEKS before her due date to reduce the shedding of parasite eggs that can contaminate the foal during his first weeks of life.

Have your foaling stall prepared. If you are almost positive of not expecting any foaling problems and the weather is going to be perfect, nature provides an excellent foaling stall under the stars. However, if it is going to be either wet or cold, the foaling should take place inside. Newborn foals are incapable of internally regulating their temperature for up to 72 hours. Cold or heat extremes place a serious stress on the foal and could result in a serious illness. Your foaling stall should have good lighting (in case of emergency), well ventilated and free of dust and drafts. Water buckets should be hung at least one foot above the floor - babies don't see real well and their coordination leaves a lot to be desired. A layer of good clean straw makes an excellent bedding for the foaling stall.

3 WEEKS BEFORE

Jennets will begin to milk up from 3 to 5 weeks before foaling. You should familiarize yourself with the jennet's mammary gland and teats. Within 24 to 48 hours of foaling, they will engorge with milk and you will be able to tell the difference.

2 TO 3 DAYS BEFORE FOALING

There is a 50/50 chance that the jennet will secrete a yellowish wax from the teats that is the forerunner to milk production. If she is actually dripping milk, you should call your vet as she may be loosing precious colostrum.

1 DAY TO 12 HOURS

If it is evening and her udder is as large as it was that same morning, close observation is warranted. She will begin to act very restless, walking from one side of the pasture to the other. She may stop eating and drinking and may also exhibit patchy sweating. A sure sign is her walking off to stand by herself and keeping a definite distance from other animals.

1 HOUR TO FOALING

She will carry her tail somewhat elevated with flicking movements which is a reflection of internal pressures. If you are keeping a very close eye on her, approximately two hours before foaling, you will notice her urinating about every 15 minutes. She may have a bout or two of diarrhea.

At the time of foaling, she will lay down, get right back up, move around, and lay back down. When the fetus enters the birth canal, it ruptures the placenta which causes her to expel a great amount of water. At this point, if you see no part of a foal within 15 minutes, call your vet immediately and keep her on her feet and walking until the vet arrives. She will give 3 or 4 strong pushes followed by a short rest. When she lies down, she will extend all four legs in a stiff manner.

At this point, you will see a grayish-white sac enclosing a forefoot, begin to appear. As long as the foal continues to come out a little with each push, everything is fine. Unless you are extremely familiar with the foaling process, pulling a foal is dangerous and could activate a too rapid delivery severely damaging both the foal and the mother.

When the shoulders are out (not before!), many foals are still encased in membrane. If this is the case and the foal kicks and breaks part of the membrane, you should step in and clear the membrane away from the foals nostrils. Once you see the foal take their first breath, grab the nose of the foal, point it toward the ground and shake it lightly to help remove excess fluid in the nostrils. The mother may or may not rest a minute to prepare for the final passage of the rump. Once this is completed, the hind legs usually slip right out. If the air temperature is cool, you may rub the foal with towels to help dry it off. This also helps stimulate respiration and circulation.

Warning: Do not sell tickets to the foaling. Jennets can become defensive and delay foaling or worse, divert their attention from the newborn. The equine's ability to control or delay, is the main reason most foals are born at night!

Chapter 4

The Foaling Process

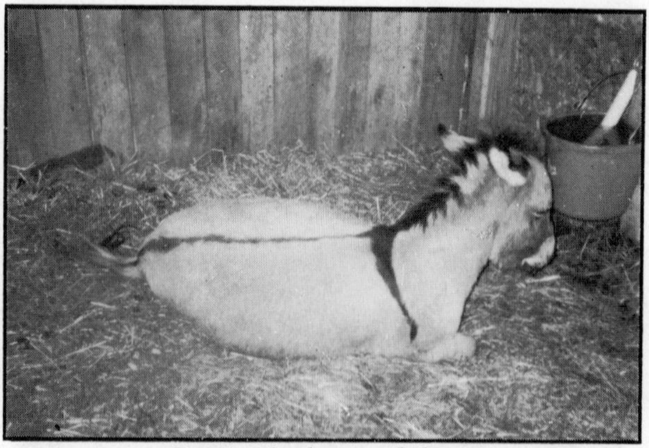

Jennet in heavy labor

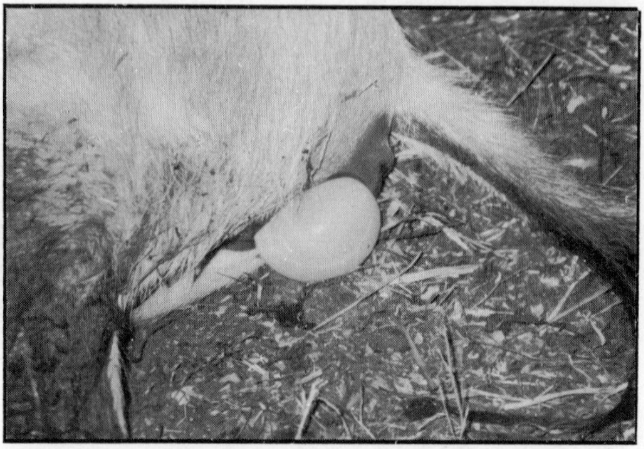

First appearance of sac

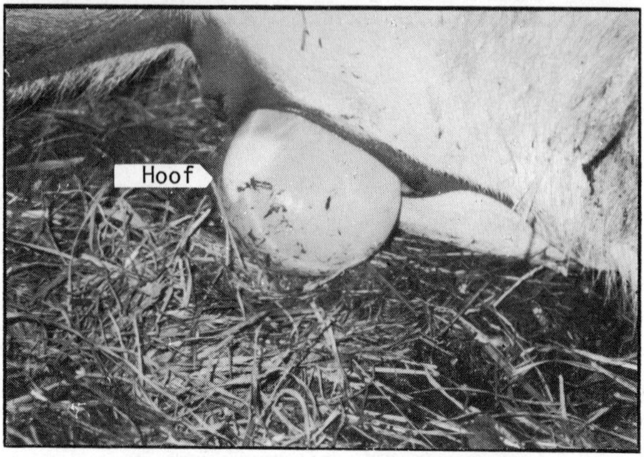

Appearance of one hoof

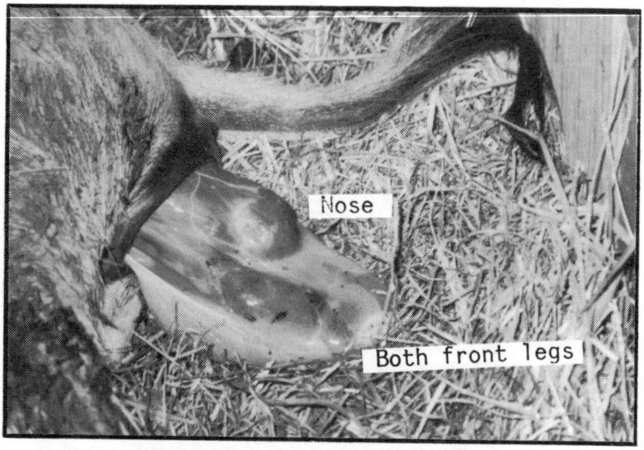

Nose and both front legs

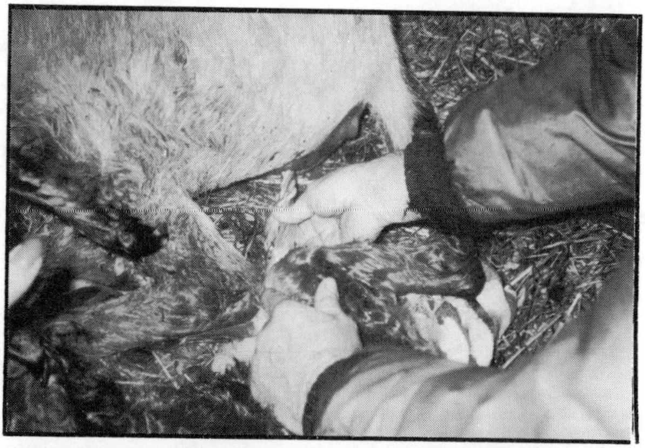

Foal still attached to umbilical cord

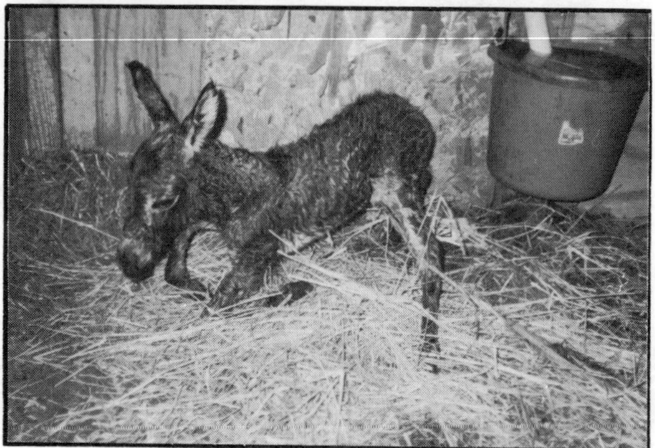

"..humm, let's try this first.."

She's In Labor!

Help! What do I do if...

(Stage One Labor)

SIGN: Jennet restless, pacing, may sweat, may pass very soft manure, roll, lie down and get up repeated.

TIME: One half hour to two hours (always keep track of time)

RED ALERT: **Jennet shows signs of severe pain, and violent rolling and thrashing on ground.**

WHAT TO DO: Call vet immediately! Make sure stall in heavily bedded with straw. Try to calm her as much as you can. If vet is on way, try to keep her on her feet.

SIGN: Stage one labor completely stops.

WHAT TO DO: Get out of the stall and out of sight. Jennets can stop Stage One labor if they are feeling too much human interference.

(Stage Two Labor)

SIGN: Contractions start. Jennet's water breaks

TIME: Usually within 2 hours of onset of Stage One of labor.

RED ALERT: **Water didn't break and you see a dark red bulge coming out.**

WHAT TO DO: Placenta Previa. Placenta's outer sac didn't rip. Call your vet and have him on the way. In mean time, you must pull foal out immediately to save him. Cut red sack, reach in and grab hold of front legs, making sure to keep legs one in front of the other. If you pull legs out evenly, he could get shoulder locked. Pull downward toward jennets back hocks - not straight out.

SIGN: Jennet starts eating hay and seems uninterested in delivering a baby.

RED ALERT: **Water broke but 15-20 minutes have passed and nothing is happening.**

WHAT TO DO: If leg is sticking out, tug on it slightly. A live foal should tug back. Oxytocin hormone is slow in being released and slight tugs on foals legs should start contractions back.
SIGN: Two foal hooves appear, positioned with soles facing downward toward jennet's hocks.

TIME: Hooves should appear within 5 minutes of water breaking.

RED ALERT: **Instead of seeing two front legs and a muzzle, you only count one leg and muzzle or no muzzle. Foal could have one leg or head bent back and you need to reach into jennet and position correctly.**

WHAT TO DO: Call your vet immediately and have him talk you through it.

SIGN: Both front legs of foal are coming out evenly and jennet stops pushing the way she should because of pain.

RED ALERT: **Either foal is being born that way or you have pulled both legs out evenly.**

WHAT TO DO: Gently pull on one leg until its situated 3 to 4 inches ahead of the other one to allow shoulders to pass.

SIGN: Jennet has pushed head and shoulders out but is getting no further.

RED ALERT: **Foal is probably "hip-locked". Get your vet on the line to help you. Grasp foal's torso and rock it gently down toward the left then down toward the right to help dislodge foal.**

(Stage Three Labor)

SIGN: Jennet has delivered foal and lays on her side resting.

WHAT TO DO: Foal's back legs are probably still inside jennet. Any movements by you should be very slow and quiet. Gently pull back legs out if you are in foaling area. Point foal's head downward and gently shake sideways to remove excess fluid from nose.

SIGN: Immediately after delivering hips, jennet jumps to her feet breaking umbilical cord.

RED ALERT: **Foal's umbilical stump bleeds heavily.**

WHAT TO DO: Immediately pinch stump to stop bleeding. Keep pinched for a minute to see if blood clots. If not, take a piece of bailing twine or thick string and tie off. Make certain bleeding has stopped. Iodine cord. It is very seldom that problems arise from cords severing too quickly, so no need to worry about loss of transfer of blood from jennet to foal. It is preferred that jennet remains still for at least two minutes, giving foal additional blood and a quicker start on life.

SIGN: When jennet stands after delivering, cord does not break and afterbirth comes out of jennet and remains attached to cord and attached to foal.

WHAT TO DO: Grab cord a minimum of one inch from foal's belly and with other hand, grab cord about six inches from foal's belly and pull hard to break cord. If stump continues to bleed, tie off. Iodine cord.

Now is the time to get out of the stall and leave mother and new baby alone!

SIGN: After standing, jennet is acting very nervous.

RED ALERT: **Jennet is either afraid of foal or attacks foal.**

WHAT TO DO: Generally this is due to 1) it is a jennet's first foal and she's unsure of what to do or 2) too much human interference. If she simply acts afraid of foal, leave them alone. If she tries to attack foal, jump in between them and do not let her near foal. Make sure jennet is haltered. Tie her up securely. Bring foal to her head and lay on ground. Talk to jennet softly and pet her or scratch her chest. Let her smell foal but make sure she can't stump with front legs. Continue to reassure her. If foal arises and she tries to kick foal, hobble her back legs. If you do not have hobbles available, tie her back legs together around the fetlock area with a T-shirt leaving about 6" in-between legs. (Enough for her to barely be able to walk, but close enough where if she kicks, she cannot kick hard enough to come in contact with foal.) Untie jennet and try leaving them alone again. If she tries to bite foal, muzzle jennet. After she is muzzled and hobbled, get out of stall and leave them alone for at least two hours before further interference by you.

SIGN: Afterbirth is hanging out of jennet. You should pick up the part that is dragging on the ground and tie it up to the rest of the afterbirth so that it does not drag ground. Additional weight will help jennet expel it.

RED ALERT: **After two hours, jennet has not expelled afterbirth.**
WHAT TO DO: Summon your vet. If contractions have stopped, he will

need to give jennet oxytocin to help her expel afterbirth.

SIGN: Two hours after birth, foal is still lying on ground.

RED ALERT: **Foal needs to nurse within 3 hours to get colostrum and nursing will give him strength.**

WHAT TO DO: Call your vet especially if foal appears to be weak.

Trouble Signs During Foaling

Trouble signs are as follows: The second stage of labor (contractions) lasting longer than 30 minutes; abnormal distress on the part of the mother; failure of the front feet and nose to appear; presence of the back feet coming first (hoof pads will face upward). Any of these signs requires immediate veterinary attention. The longer the jennet is in labor, the more difficult the birth process is for the foal. Another problem associated with prolonged labor is a dry birth canal. The fluid that is released at the end of the first stage of labor lubricates the foal's passageway, but if expulsion of the foal is delayed, the birth canal may become very dry, making labor even more difficult. In these cases, mineral oil is sometimes used for lubrication so that the foal can slip through the birth canal.

If your vet is on his way, get the mother up and walking. This helps to reduce the force of the contractions and, in many instances, allows the foal to drop back into the uterus. This can delay parturition for 30 to 60 minutes. Sometimes veterinary help is difficult to get hold of or possibly they live quite a distance from you. There are times when you must take matters into your own hands.

A breech birth is very serious and requires immediate assistance. This foal must be delivered within minutes as the foal's blood supply is compromised and also the cord may be severed before the head and shoulders arrive. In a breech birth, you will see the back hocks coming out instead of the nose. You must help the mother by grabbing the back legs above the fetlock (ankle) and pulling. IMPORTANT: Do NOT pull the foal out straight - pull toward the mother's back heels - downward.

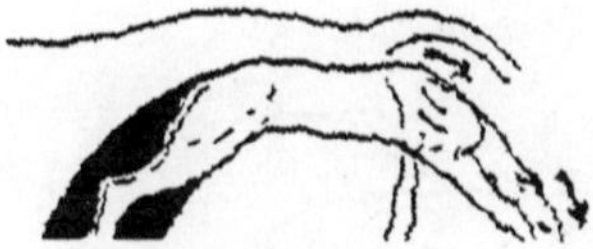

If the jennet must be aided, traction on the foal should follow an arc out and down toward the mother's hocks.

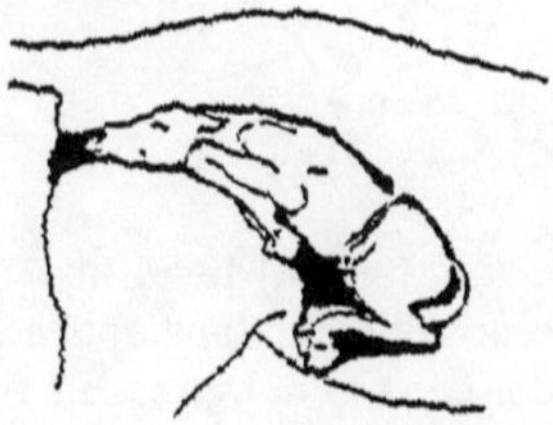

One or both forelegs folded under. Push foal back into uterus and extend legs in correct position. While handling legs, be gentle so that you do not damage uterine wall with foal's foot.

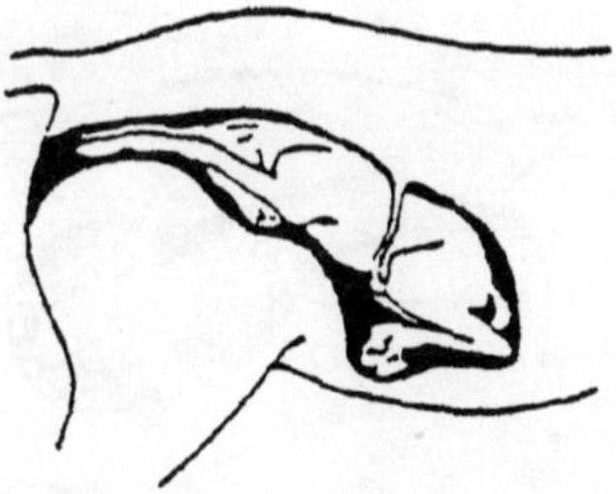

When the foal's nose is not found in the birth canal, it may be found tucked downward. The foal must be pushed back and head lifted.

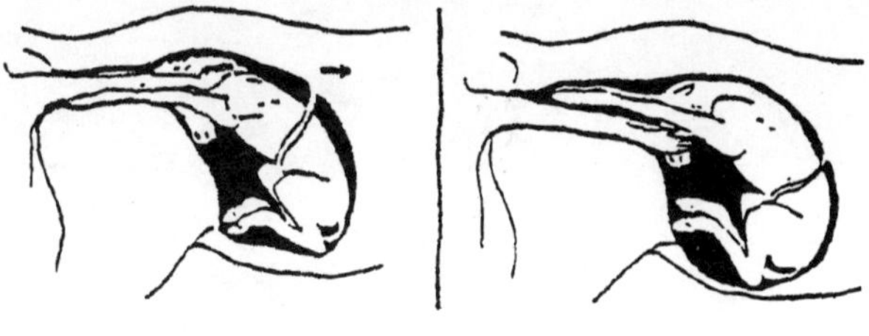

In order to correct many abnormal positions:
(A) Foal is gently pressed back into the uterus to obtain working room for manipulation.
(B) The misplaced portion of foal (in this instance the head) is placed in the normal position for delivery.
(C) The foal is guided into the birth canal.

(A) (B)

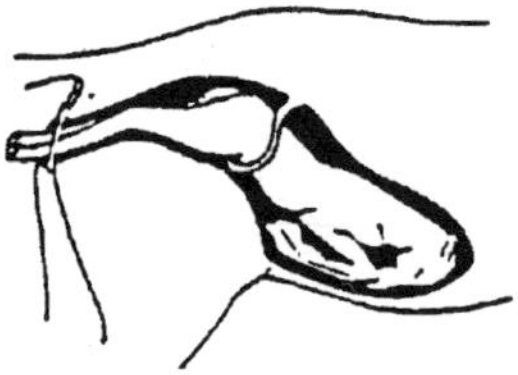

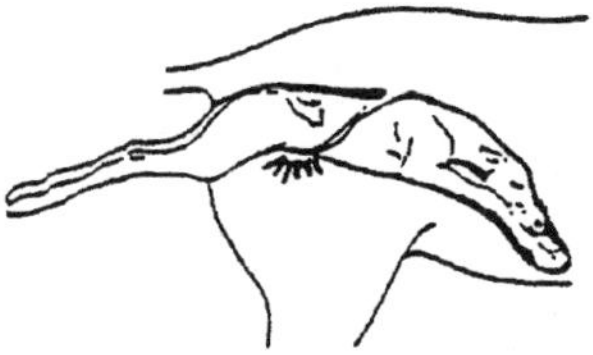

(A) The first two joints of the hind leg (hock & fetlock) bend in opposite directions. In this manner the true backward position can be identified.
(B) In backward position the foal's umbilical cord is compressed against the pelvic. This can cause suffocation if delivery does not proceed quickly.

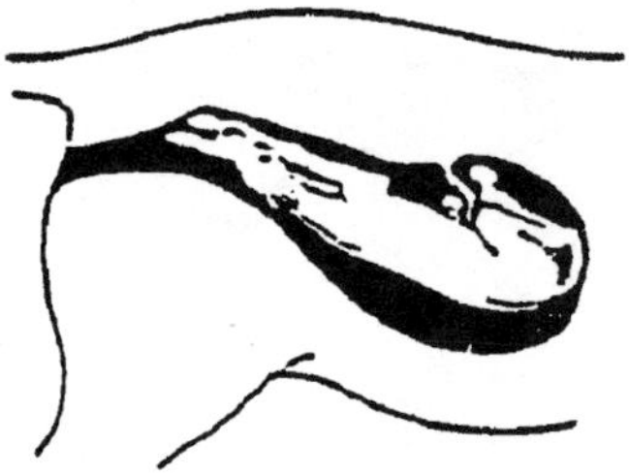

When present in this position, the arch of the foal's back does not complement the upward curve of the birth canal. Before delivery, foal must be repositioned by rotation.

Should You Help Pull That Foal Out?

Dystocia: *Is the term applied to any type of abnormal or difficult birth which prevents the jennet from delivering a foal by her own efforts.*

You're panicked, the jennet has been in labor for quite some time, and you have no baby. Most of you call me much too long after the labor began to save the foal. Jennets do not stay in labor for hours (or days) like humans do. It's a fairly rapid process and you have a very limited amount of time to make decisions. This is being written in layman's language - no fancy words - so that you understand exactly what you are looking for, and not wondering what a certain word means.

Always time the sequence of events.

I always make note of the time I see the jennet go into labor. Most jennets will begin acting very nervous and most will have one or two streams of diarrhea. This nervousness can last 5 minutes, or I believe the longest I've noticed, is two hours. When I see the first contraction (the jennet will still be standing), I begin the countdown. Within 15 to 20 minutes of that first contraction, I want to see some action, in the way of her laying down and pushing.

From the time of the first contraction, I want to see the foal's hooves and a nose within 45 minutes.

If I don't, I place a call to my veterinarian. I want him on the line so that I can say "get here as fast as you can", if need be. If you do not see a nose and hooves within that 45 minute time frame, you probably have a problem. Now again, don't panic. It may be a very simple problem such as a bent back hoof or something else that is fairly easy to solve.

Now, before we get started with the rest of this article, I want to give you some advice. Read this article at least four times. Imprint it in your brain. You will be absolutely amazed at what will come back to you in an emergency when any other time you couldn't remember this stuff if your life depended on it. Years ago I was sitting on the ground playing with a month old jennet. She apparently had something in her mouth and while she was crawling over my body, it became lodged in her throat. She fell over on the ground and wasn't breathing. I picked her up behind her front legs and performed the heimlich maneuver and she began breathing again and was fine. I sat on the ground shaking, wondering how in the world I knew to immediately do this. I apparently read it somewhere and it just came to me. Now, back to our original subject.

Once the jennet's water breaks, you should see a white sac within 5 to 10 minutes.

If the jennet's water breaks and she gets up and walks around, it make take a little longer for the white sac to appear. Again, time is of the essence.

Any prolonged foaling could result in the foal not getting the external oxygen supply that he needs because the placenta has detached or the umbilical cord in being pinched inside the birth canal.

You see the nose and front legs but nothing else is happening. The nose and legs are sticking out and the jennet is pushing, but 15 minutes later, things have not changed. The foal has remained in this position. Why isn't the foal coming out? Sometimes maiden jennets will only give half pushes because when they push hard, it hurts. Maybe the pelvic opening is not large enough. Maybe the foal is not in the correct position and its shoulders are stuck. The longer you wait, the drier the birth canal gets, and the harder it is to pull the foal out. If some time has passed since the water broke, put on a plastic glove and squirt mineral oil all over it, slide your hand just inside the birth canal on the sides of the foal and lubricate.

45 Minutes after first contraction and either there is no sign of the foal or, the nose and legs have remained stationary. Telephone your vet and have him advise you. Tell him <u>exactly</u> what you see and what has happened. Tell him <u>exactly</u> what parts of the foal you can see (if any) and <u>exactly</u> what position those parts are in. If your vet can get to you within 15 minutes, he may advise you to keep the jennet standing and walking to prevent the foal from twisting or coming out any further and it may also drop the foal back into the uterus giving him more room to manipulate a foal that is not in the correct birthing position. This will again depend on exactly what has happened up to this point in time.

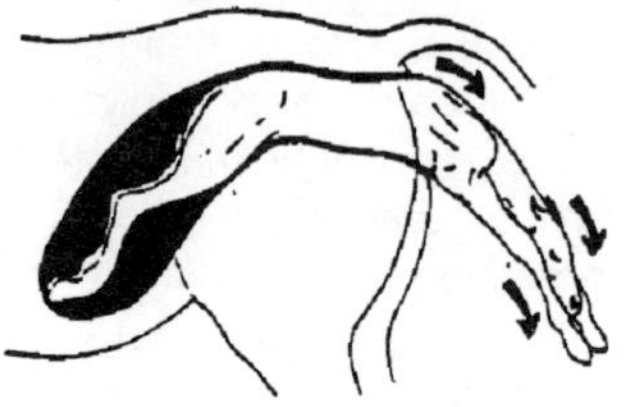

Correct Position of Foal during Birth

If you see a bright red sac protruding from the jennet, you have a case of placenta previa. This is premature separation of the placenta and is an emergency. Unless this red membrane is opened and the foal's head exposed promptly, the foal will suffocate. Cut this red sac with a pair of scissors if you cannot rip it open. Follow the directions for pulling the foal out - later in this article. (If you cannot find the foal's legs and head, the foal is not in the correct foaling position.)

Above is the correction position of the foal.

1) The first thing you will see is the white sac with a white hoof inside it. Approximately 2" to 3" behind that will be another white hoof. Another 2" beyond that will be the nose of the foal.

2) First appearance of hooves and legs: In the correct position, the legs will be side by side or one slightly on top of the other. They should not be coming out evenly. One leg slightly behind the other also means that the large shoulders will be coming out at an angle making it easier to get through the pelvis area.

3) Nearest the tail, will be the nose of the foal.

Any deviation from the position of the above photo means the foal in not in the correct birthing position.

The above photo shows exactly where most jennets - if they are having a difficult time getting the foal out - will get stuck. The jennet has not dilated enough, the front feet may be coming out evenly and the shoulders are stuck, or a maiden jennet is just too tight to push the foal out any further.

When the decision has been made that the jennet needs help in getting this foal out, this is what you need to do. It's very simple.
Take both hands and wrap them around the front legs up to where the end of the nose is. When the jennet pushes, you pull. DO NOT pull one leg out further than the other. Grab BOTH legs just as they are (one out further than the other) and pull evenly on both legs. If that foal is stuck, don't think a little tug is all that's needed. You are going to have to really pull. If the jennet stops her contractions, give a slight pull on the legs. This will usually make her have a contraction and push.

Important: Never pull straight out. Remember, the foal in at an angle in the birth canal. You have to pull down towards the jennets back legs at that same angle.

Don't let go of the legs. Keep pulling whenever the jennet pushes until the foal is out. Remove the sac from the nose of the foal immediately.

Oh No! The nose and legs are out and the jennet jumps up while I was pulling and now she's standing!

Don't panic and don't let go. Keep pulling downward. You may have to follow the jennet around if she starts walking. Keep pulling. Hopefully someone else is there with you who can grab the jennet's head and keep her still if she starts walking. If you have to pull a foal out when the jennet is standing, sometimes the afterbirth will come out with the foal and sometimes it will stay in and the cord will break prematurely. If the cord breaks prematurely, you will see a lot of blood. Don't be too concerned. If the cord is bleeding from the foal's side, clamp it with your fingers then tie it with a heavy string and iodine. If it isn't bleeding from the foal's side, just iodine it. We have had probably 10 cords break prematurely and have never had a problem with the foal losing that additional blood.

If you followed the above instructions, and the foal was in the correct foaling position to begin with, you should now have a live foal on the ground. Pay particular attention to the time frames in this article. Most of the time, after you see the first contraction, you will have a baby on the ground within one hour. I have no idea how many foals Mike and I have saved by helping to pull the baby out. I do know that my records indicate at least 20 foals (out of around 250) could ***not*** have been delivered without assistance.

Abnormal Foal Positions

The above covers foals that are in the ***correct*** birthing position, it's just that they were stuck and could not have been born without their owners assistance.

There are times that a jennet goes into labor, has contractions, and either the wrong body part is coming out at the wrong time or no body parts are coming out. When you have your vet on the phone, he may ask you to stick your hand inside the jennet and try to determine exactly what it is you are feeling. Your first thought is "Oh Lord, I can't do this". Well, if you have an emergency, the Lord says you CAN and WILL do this. Take a few deep breaths, calm down, put a plastic glove on, with some mineral oil or OB lubricant, and go to work. This isn't going to bother or hurt your jennet. Your hand is a lot smaller than what she has been trying to push out. It can be difficult to figure out what you are feeling. Look at the following drawings and compare them to what you feel and try to figure it out. My belief is that it is very difficult to reposition a mal-positioned foal in a miniature. There just isn't enough room. In horse mares, you have the room to push a foal back into the uterus and do a lot of rearranging. However, if you just have a bent back leg, a bent back hoof or shoulders coming out too straight, you certainly can correct these and get the baby out - alive.

Dystocia

The definition of dystocia is an abnormal or difficult birth. A very difficult birth, a prolonged birth along with the necessity of cesarean section or prolapse, all fall under the category of dystocia. Dystocia will in all likelihood not let your jennet be a candidate for rebreeding for at least four months due to the inflammation associated with the healing process.

Along with inflammation, injured tissues experience heat and swelling and the production of pus. If all goes well, the debris is drained out and does not accumulate and the rebuilding process in the uterus takes place. If drainage is impaired and accumulates inside the body, more damage occurs naturally and through the intervention by man to drain the infection.

Sperm will not survive in an inflamed uterus. Heat kills sperm and the general swelling stops the sperm from continuing their journey. In additional, the bodies natural defenses look upon the sperm as intruders which the body's antibodies quickly kill.

In severe cases, damage to the cervix can prevent a jennet from ever conceiving again. The cervix must be able to close tightly to prevent outside contamination from entering - thus killing the fetus. It must also be able to relax itself enough to allow passage of a foal.

If a jennet has dystocia, sufficient time should be allowed for the reproductive tract to heal itself. Damage to the reproductive tract can even occur in what you might perceive as an "easy foaling", however, if you did have a jennet who had a difficult foaling and you cannot get her rebred, this should be one of the first things you mention to your vet.

Sometimes more difficult signs can be missed such as a creamy appearance to the allantoic fluid (when the jennet's water breaks) instead of a clear "tea" color, a placenta that has one or more patchy areas of discoloration, or a placenta that was retained more than two hours - which could happen if the jennet foaled when no one was around.

Clues like these indicate the placenta may have become infected during the later stages of pregnancy and are certainly things your vet needs to know.

Summary:

I think that in a great many instances, jennets are not ready to breed back in their foal heats and much damage can be done to the reproductive tract when it has not had time to heal from the trauma of giving birth. The jack can cause additional inflammation and admit unneeded bacteria. Some jennets just simply need a longer period of time for the reproductive tract to cleanse itself.

The pain of a still swollen uterus is something that a jennet may not forgot and associate being with a jack as causing pain, hence causing jennets to become difficult breeders.

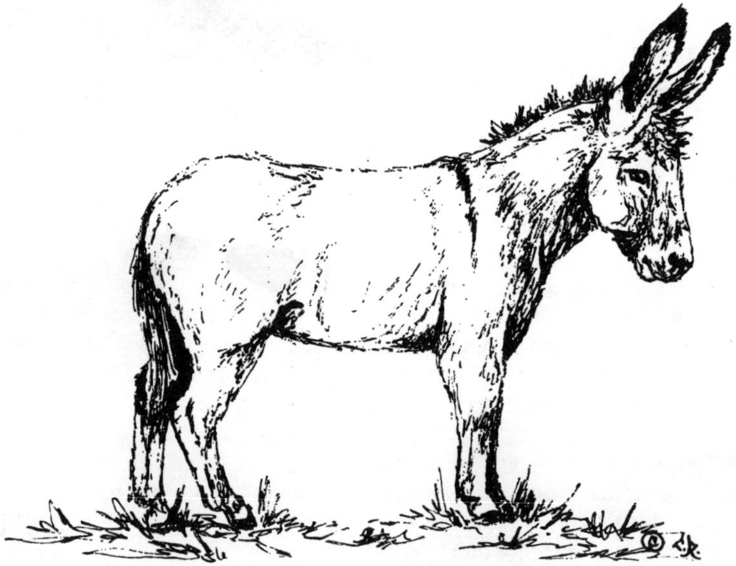

Chapter 5

Jennet Aftercare

Expulsion of the Afterbirth

Often the membranes are passed with the foal. If not, expulsion normally takes place from 10 minutes to 4 hours. The placenta may be red, brown or purplish in color. During this period uterine contractions continue and the jennet will show signs of discomfort. These contractions continue after foaling and help cleanse the tract of fluid and debris and return the expanded uterus to its normal size.

If you have to call your vet for any reason, one of the first things he will usually ask to examine when he arrives is the placenta. The vet will want to determine if it is all there or if there are pieces missing. Their condition will tell him much about the condition of the mother's uterus. Once expulsion takes place, remove them and place them in a bucket of water. Put them in a place where no other animal can get to them and keep them for at least 24 hours.

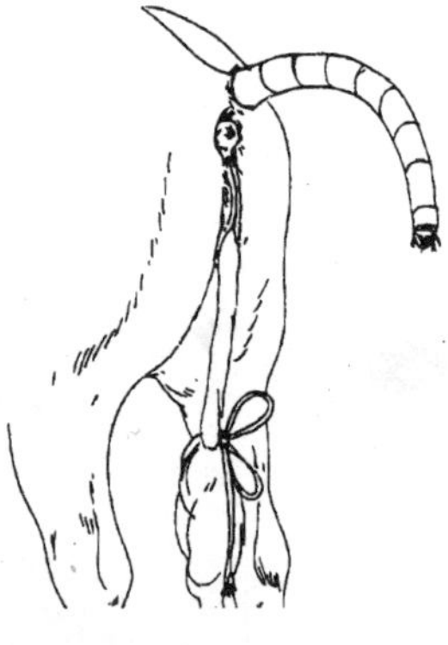

The jennet should pass the membranes within one or two hours if everything is proceeding normally. They are considered retained if they stay in her beyond three hours. If portions are hanging out of her vulva, DO NOT CUT THEM! Their weight helps to pull the rest of the placenta loose. Instead of letting the membrane drag the ground, tie it up with a piece of baling twine. Doing this helps add weight to it and helps the jennet expel it easier. Never attempt to pull the membranes out.

Most vets prefer that you call them if the membranes have not passed in about three hours. The donkey is then given penicillin or other antibiotic treatment for three days, especially if there is any sign of infection. The vet may also put an antibiotic solution into the uterus to help flush it out and kill any infection which is present. If the membranes are left in place for more than about 8 hours after foaling, the donkey may develop a laminitis or make her founder - an extremely serious problem.

UNSEEN DANGER - The Retained Placenta

Your jennet has just foaled, but she has not yet shed her placenta. How long should you wait before you become concerned and call your veterinarian? This can vary a bit, depending on the situation. It helps to know some things about the placental membranes - the important tissues that serve as life-support systems for the fetus.

As soon as labor begins, the placenta starts its process of detachment, especially during second stage labor, when the foal is being expelled. In most normal births, the placenta is still sufficiently attached to supply the foal during the birth process, but there are some instances in which the placenta detaches too early and comes out ahead of or with, the foal. In these cases the foal will die unless the birth is accomplished swiftly. *(Refer to placenta previa in this book.)*

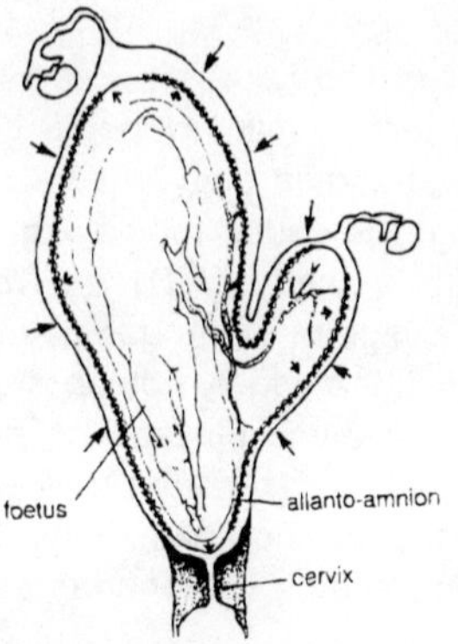

Contraction of uterus increases pressure on membranes. This forces membranes through the only distensible region - the cervix.

In most births, the placenta remains somewhat attached until after the foal is born and the uterus goes through another series of contractions as it sheds the placenta and begins shrinking. Many jennets shed the placenta within 20 to 30 minutes after foaling. They lie there for a time after the birth, resting (and the umbilical cord is still pulsing, pumping blood into the foal - some of the foal's blood supply is within the placenta but will drain into the foal if jennet and foal are allowed to lie there a few minutes before the cord is broken). Then the mare will get up, 15 to 30 minutes after the birth, and at this time the cord will break and the placenta will be seen hanging down from the vulva. Many mares will shed it as they get up; the membranes fall out of the vagina at this time.

But if a jennet is upset and gets up too quickly, problems can result. The cord will be broken too soon, depriving the foal of blood, and the placenta that was starting to detach and work its way through the birth canal may fall back into the uterus as the jennet gets up. The uterus and cervix are starting to contract, and it may be harder to expel the placenta if the cervix is starting to close and the placenta has fallen back into the uterus.

If the placenta is hanging down and dragging, tie it into a ball or knot about level with the jennet's hocks or a little higher, to keep her or the foal from stepping on it and tearing it. This will also keep it from bumping or dragging against the jennet's hind legs, which might startle her or cause her to kick at it (and possibly injure the foal). The weight of the ball will help keep gentle tension and ease the membranes on out after a time. You don't want the dragging placenta to be stepped on or forcibly pulled, or it may tear off inside the mare, leaving a piece in the uterus, to cause infection.

The placenta starts to decompose rapidly after the birth of the foal, and if any of it is left inside, it creates an ideal place for infection. Thus it is important to check it for completeness once it is shed. Spread out on the ground, it should look like a pair of trousers with the ends of the legs closed. The only tear should be at the "waist", where the foal came through. Usually, if any part is missing, it will be one of the tips of the "legs"'.

Most jennets shed the placenta within one-half to two hours; it is unusual for a jennet to take longer than three or four hours. Anything longer than three hours should be cause for worry and you should call your vet. A placenta retained for six to eight hours or longer is cause for having the jennet thoroughly checked, even if the placenta is shed. (*MDT Ed Note*: Richard Linhart, D.V.M., Diplomat, American College of Theriogenologists, Kentucky tells us, "By definition, a mare/jennet that does not pass the placenta within 3 hours after giving birth has a retained placenta. There are several possible side affects or sequela to a retained placenta including: founder, septic metritis (uterine infections) and colic. Given the severity of these conditions, jennets should be seen by a veterinarian soon after this 3 hour period.")

Never try to help a mare shed her placenta. Even gentle pulling can cause bleeding or tearing. If the placenta tears apart, tie the broken off piece back to the rest of it and leave it in a knot to give weight to the mass to help it work on out.

The veterinarian can tell a lot about the health of the placenta (and mare and foal) by the appearance of the shed membranes. A fresh, healthy placenta should be bright-red to red-brown, with a velvety look. If off-color, it could be inspected.

Retained placenta is fairly common following a difficult foaling (especially if the jennet had to have assistance), birth of twins, or induced labor. A few less common causes are birth of a premature foal, or dietary imbalance such as lack of phosphorus.

In treating a retained placenta, the veterinarian may give the jennet an IV injection of oxytocin to stimulate contraction of the uterus and hasten expulsion. He may start the jennet on antibiotics, or flush or irrigate the uterus in an attempt to gently remove any small tags of placental membrane that might still be inside, put antibiotic boluses into the uterus, or pump in a liquid antibiotic.

Any time the placenta is retained, you can suspect some degree of infection. It may be temporary and local, or become systemic and life-threatening. A localized infection may damage the uterus, causing problems with future fertility (leaving fibrous scar tissue that may interfere with future conception or inhibit blood supply to the fetus during the next pregnancy).

If infection gets beyond the uterus and into the bloodstream, it can become fatal. The jennet becomes obviously sick, with high temperature, depression, lack of appetite and decrease in milk. The infection may lead to laminitis (foaling founder), in which the jennet will be very lame. If this condition isn't treated immediately, she may die or be permanently crippled.

Therefore, jennets should be closely watched after the birth, especially if the placenta was retained. A temperature check twice daily can give clues about her health. Any fever, lateness in passing the placenta, lameness, signs of colic, or loss of interest in feed, or decrease in milk flow (the foal not getting enough, always hungry) during the first few days after foaling should be a signal to call your vet, as a medical emergency. Thus the final stage of labor is just as crucial as the foaling. If there is trouble, you will be more able to get medical assistance in time to head off a disaster.

Reference: Written by Heather Smith-Thomas

UNDERSTANDING MILK PRODUCTION

The jennet's udder is located between her hind legs and is arranged in two halves. Each half of the udder is composed of two glands and each gland has a separate drainage network although they are supplied by common nerves and blood vessels.

During lactation (the period of milk production), each gland contains a collection of tiny, sac-like cavities (alveoli) which are lined with special milk-producing cells. This milk-producing unit is surrounded by a connective tissue referred to as a lobule. Ducts from each lobule drain into the teat cisterns which supply each teat canal. The teat opening is closed by a muscle which normally prevents milk from streaming out of the teat until milk ejection is stimulated.

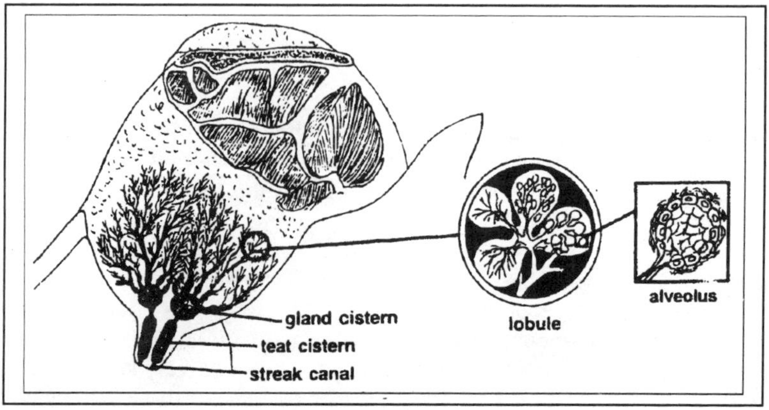

Although milk production is initiated during pregnancy, the release of milk from the alveoli is normally inhibited until just prior to or just after foaling. Researchers have suggested that high levels of estrogen and progesterone during pregnancy stimulates the release of prolactin (a hormone that stimulates milk secretion).

Retention of milk prior to foaling swells the alveoli and depresses milk production. Release of the hormone oxytocin during foaling causes contractions of the cells in the alveoli and causes milk let-down. Frequent suckling or manual milking enhances milk production.

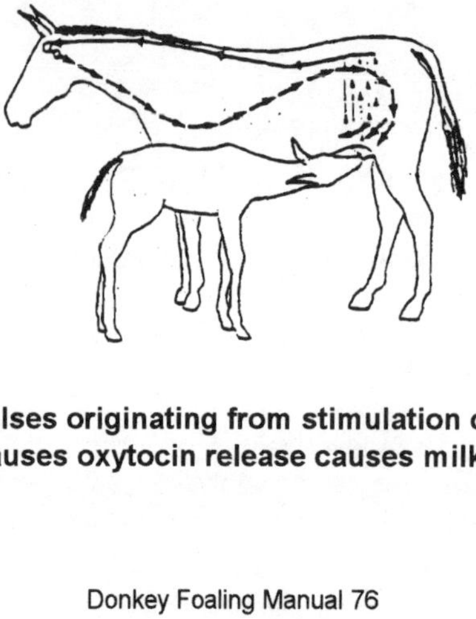

Nerve impulses originating from stimulation of the teats nursing causes oxytocin release causes milk let-down

When the mammary gland produces milk but is not suckled or milked, as happens during late pregnancy, a yellowish, slightly syrupy milk is produced. This milk is called colostrum and contains high levels of vitamins, minerals, proteins and fat. It also contains elements which have a laxative effect on the foal's digestive system and antibodies which establish passive immunity within the foal's bloodstream for the first few months of life.

As long as the foal nurses, stimulation of the nerve endings in the teats triggers the release of hormones that produce milk.

Care of the Jennet after Foaling

Unless disturbed, the jennet will usually lay quietly immediately after the birth for up to 20 minutes. During this time the jennet will frequently lift her head to check on her foal. This is the most critical period for the development of a strong bond between the jennet and her foal. The smell of the fetal membranes seems to play some role in the jennet's identification and acceptance of her foal. Certain procedures should be carried out immediately after foaling, however, human intervention should be minimal during the first two hours.

This is the time to double check your stall to make certain it has been "foal proofed". There will be numerous falls by the foal until they get on their feet and manage to stay there.

If the weather is cold, you should have turned the heat lamps on in the stall as soon as the jennet went into labor. If you haven't done that, you should do so. You may also want to quickly rub the foal down with a towel, if the weather is cold.

Offer the jennet a bucket of lukewarm, not cold, water. An hour or two after foaling you may want to offer her a little grain. Now leave the two alone and if you must, watch through a peephole in the stall. DO NOT invite all the neighbors over to see the new baby!

You will want to keep the jennet and newborn in a stall by themselves for this first night. Weather permitting, you can leave them out in a pasture the next day. We generally leave the two out in our foaling pasture for an hour or two at a time for the first 2 days. We take them out and put them in probably four or five times a day until the foals legs have gained strength. Jennets are extremely protective at this time and the foal may get injured on weak legs in the midst of all the fuss being made over him.

So What Happens After the Delivery?

Recovery And Discovery

The mysterious hormonal storm that ended pregnancy and orchestrated delivery gently rolls away. The swelling of the jennet's legs and belly subsides, and while she may still be a bit stiff and sore, especially around her hind end, she becomes much more active.

In a process called involution, the uterus continues to contract for some days after birth. This rids the organ of the excess exudate and fluids that accompany pregnancy and birth, and enables the uterus to decease in an accordion-like fashion, with its wall pleating, compressing and folding in on itself.

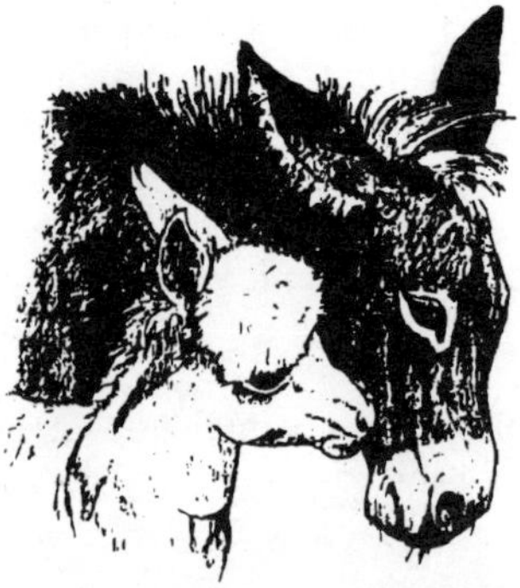

The jennet's attention is sharply focused on protecting and nurturing her foal. She is constantly by his side, standing over him when he sleeps and defending him against intrusions and disturbances. These maternal urges are both instinctive and learned. In the wild, mares who didn't defend their foals soon lost them.

For his part, the foal rapidly gains strength and vigor. His respiration is still fast but his temperature stabilizes. Early in the first day, the foal passes the meconium, or first stool, which appears as rubbery, dark-colored lumps. Squatting and straining will be common stances as he urinates and defecates frequently, though the amount of urine varies. The feces are mustard colored and less solid, reflecting the content of his diet.

Significant internal changes are also occurring during the first day of the foal's life. Early on, a hole in the foal's head, known as the ductus arteriosus, will close. In the womb, this hole connected the foal's pulmonary artery to the aorta, bypassing the usual route of blood flow through the lungs since they were not yet operational. The foal's eyesight is quickly corning on line, though he still has little awareness of anything but his physical needs.

As the jennet caters to her growing youngster, her body is undergoing change as well. Within a week following parturition, minor injuries of the birth canal have healed. The vulva has contracted and muscle tone has returned to the pelvic area, eliminating the sunken appearance around the tail head. The uterus has almost completed its involution and is by now about 1½ times its prepregnancy size. The jennet is no longer sore and resumes social relations with her herdmates. Her milk production has not yet reached full capacity, which it will when the foal's milk demands peak in about three weeks.

Inside, the jennet's system is gearing up to sustain another new life. She enters an estrous cycle, called "foal heat," and if bred, the new egg produced within her ovary can be fertilized. If the jennet is a bit slow to return to normal, this abbreviated heat cycle further tones the uterus, opens the cervix for temporary drainage and helps the reproductive system finish its cleanup job.

During the first week of his life, the foal's sense of adventure and his curiosity for things apart from himself increase dramatically. He is now socially aware of other donkeys, including his newborn peers, and develops an understanding of danger and an awareness that hazards exist.

He doesn't gain much weight or height during this first week. Instead, his energy is funneled into further refinement and improvement of body systems, organs and structures, and his coordination and muscle tone improve daily. It is not unusual to see him eat adult manure. This actually increases the presence of beneficial rnicro-organisms within his intestines, helping to "inoculate" his digestive tract and aid in food digestion.

The Fork In The Road

By the time her foal is one month old, the jennet is producing as much milk as she possibly can. Her udder is probably as large as it was prior to delivery.

This is also an experimental time for the foal. He puts anything and everything into his mouth as he learns to discern the edible from the inedible and the harmless from the noxious. He has little time to lose in developing his culinary tastes, for he will soon start to show interest in adult food. In a matter of months he will be weaned away from his dam, and though he may remember her if they live in close proximity, he will be more interested in his young herdmates than in her.

This is as it should be, because if the jennet was not rebred on foal heat, she is entering a second and longer heat cycle. With her uterus back to normal and even severe tears of the birth canal fully healed, she is now prepared to repeat the miraculous process that brought forth the frisky foal soon to leave her side.

Why Mares Reject Their Foals

A look at three reasons why, and what can be done about it

The birth of a foal should be a joyous occasion, but it can be spoiled if the mare rejects her newborn foal. This doesn't happen often, but it does happen.

There are three reasons that mares reject foals:

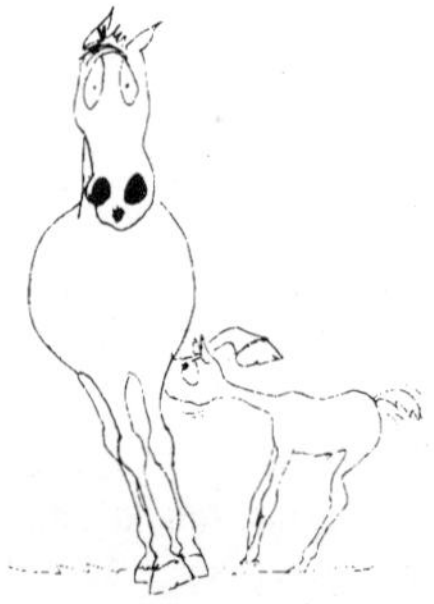

Ouch! That smarts!

1. **Painful udder**. The simplest form of foal rejection is caused by an udder that is painfully swollen. It is also the easiest to solve. In these cases, the mare doesn't actually reject the foal. In fact, she may definitely want the foal. However, she will not allow it to nurse, and if the foal is persistent in his efforts to nurse, the mare might begin to kick at the foal, or otherwise injure him.

The problem can be resolved, usually, by twitching the mare, or tranquilizing her, or hobbling either a front leg or back leg. In some cases, I have used all three options. With assistance, the foal can then nurse, relieving the pressure and edema within the udder.

More severe cases can be helped with an injection of Lasix® to relieve congestion and edema. If these methods are inadequate, the mare can be milked by hand, and the foal bottle-fed the colostrum thus obtained. I advise that, when bottle-feeding the foal, the bottle be held close to the udder so that the foal wilt seek that area for subsequent feedings once he begins to nurse.

2. **The "bad-mother" syndrome**. Sometimes, in any kind of an animal, including humans, a mother will inexplicably kill her newborn young.

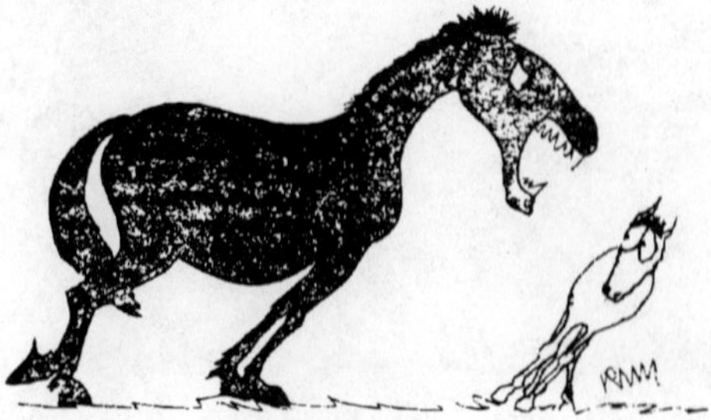

I hate it!

The cause of this is a mental aberration. It can be caused by stress, as happens often in confined zoo animals; or by behavior triggered by hormonal activity. I have seen it in horses, dogs, cats, pigs, a tiger, a leopard, and a gorilla.

When it occurs in mares, and fortunately it doesn't happen too often, the mare savages or attacks the foal, often biting him to death. In my personal experience, this behavior has occurred most often in Thoroughbred mares, but that's just my observation, not a documented statistic.

If the foal can be reached in time, the only solution here is to separate dam and foal. Sometimes the mare can be sedated, and with great caution, the foal re-introduced to the mare. Certain mares will savage every foal they bear. In other cases, it happens but once.

3. **The fearful mare**. The most common cause of foal rejection, is fear. I have read of this explanation, and that's what encouraged me to write this article. If one witnesses this kind of rejection, this is what happens: The mare foals normally. When she gets to her feet, there is this strange little creature in the stall with her. Usually the foaling has occurred in a stall, because these mares are what I call "hot-house" mares. They have spent their lives in a pampered, confined, artificial environment.

They haven't grown up on a range or in a large-pasture environment, with equine of different ages and genders and temperaments. They haven't witnessed birth and death like wild equine do in their normal environment. They react to the new foal with fear, just as they would if they have never seen a pig, or a donkey, or a sheep. If the afterbirth is hanging from their hindquarters, that panics them farther. They are already upset by the pangs of labor they have endured. Now a strange creature has suddenly appeared in their territory.

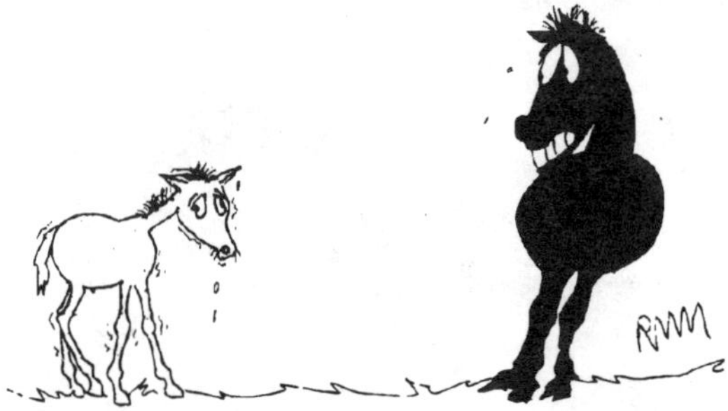

What is it?

When the foal starts to flop around, and struggles to his feet, that panics mother all the more. Then, when the foal approaches her, and she cannot escape, she freaks out and might defensively injure the foal. If she knocks it down, or kicks it away, that reinforces that behavior and she will repeat it. Often, a painful udder complicates and worsens the situation.

In order to test the validity of my theory, I telephoned two large Nebraska ranches that breed and raise purebred Arabian horses on extensive range lands. The horses breed and reproduce in pasture under conditions close to what nature intended for this species. Bill Munson, D.V.M., of the Shalimar Ranch near Harrison, Neb., told me that he has never experienced a foal rejection by a range mare, and that's out of a couple of hundred foalings. In mares kept in stalls, he did experience one mare that savaged and killed two of five foals. Tranquilizers solved that problem. Another mare, also kept in a stall, was frightened by the flopping of her placenta, and panicked and attacked her foal. Rush Creek Land and Livestock Company, Lisco, Neb., producer of famed purebred Arabian endurance-racing horses, has raised at least 900 purebred Arabian foals under range conditions. They have also produced many half-Arabians and horses of other breeds. In 1990, the ranch had its first experience with a mare rejecting a foal, and that was a mare that had never experienced any new foals in her pasture.

So, in well over a thousand foalings involving the breed most susceptible to rejecting foals, not a single mare raised in a large herd rejected her foal. The answer to the problem, then is to raise foals in many-thousand-acre pastures! Well, that isn't going to help most breeders. Not many of us, can raise horses under such conditions. There is also a down side to mares foaling unattended in very large pastures Once in a while a mare will have a foaling problem which, without human assistance, will mean the death of the foal and/or the mare.

For 25 years I have advocated the handling and manipulation of foals as soon as they were born. I call this method imprint training. I believe that imprint training of the newborn foal can prevent the third and most common type of foal rejection. I have asked hundreds of people who have imprint-trained thousands of foals, if they have ever experienced a fear-induced foal rejection. Not a single one has thus far been reported, and the majority of these mares were kept in confinement. They were not range-raised and range-bred mares. Even if a case is ultimately reported to me, its uniqueness would not alter my conclusion that imprint training at birth can prevent foal rejection.

Here is what I think happens. The mare, usually a first-foal mare, lies down, and goes into labor. She is in great discomfort. Finally, the pains stop and, exhausted, she gets to her feet. "What's this? A little, wet, weird-looking stranger in my stall? Fear! But, wait! My owner is crouched over it, touching it. Holding it down! Thank goodness! My owner is protecting me from *The Thing*!" Reassured, the mare eventually gathers the courage to approach the foal. She sniffs it. It smells very interesting. The human handling the foal has the same smell on his or her hands. Eventually, she tastes the foal. She licks it. She's hooked! From that point on, she wants it. With the presence of a human reassuring her, the mare accepts a foal that might otherwise have caused her to panic and reject it.

There's a bonus. A lot of mares, especially the next day, get very aggressive and protective of their foals. Some of them act like real tigers. I have not yet had a dam of a foal that I imprint-trained at birth show such aggression towards me. I think that the reaction of the mare is "What's this? Something threatening my baby . . . Kill! . . . But wait! He's the guy who smelled like my foal when he was born. I accepted them together. I guess he's okay." When a mare rejects a foal, analyze why she is acting that way. Is it reason No. I, 2, or 3? Or is it a combination of two of those reasons? Then, handle the problem accordingly.

Reference: Although this article was specifically written for horses, all of it can be applied to miniature donkeys. The author/illustrator, Dr. Miller, is a well known highly regarded veterinarian who has written many books and articles. He is probably most well known for his research on imprinting newborn foals. Dr. Miller is also a mule owner/lover.

FOAL REJECTION - A Donkey Breeder's Point of View

What You Can Do To Help

We usually get one or two phone calls every month from someone who feels their jennets are rejecting their newborn foals. These calls fall into one of two categories. #1 A jennet who has foaled and successfully raised a previous foal and #2 A maiden jennet who has never foaled before.

First let's cover #1. These jennets are not attacking their foals, but do not seem to want to let them nurse. When the newborn tries to nurse, the jennet will either walk away, take her nose and push the foal away or casually kick at the foal to keep it from nursing. Most of these phone calls come some three or four hours after the foal was born.

Jennets will bag up (udder becomes full of milk) anywhere from several hours to three days before foaling. Immediately after foaling, their bags and teats become engorged with milk and they will get very sore and tender. If you watch a newborn, you will see them poking their noses all over the jennet, looking for their first meal. When the newborn does this to the jennet's udder, it causes her pain.

There are a number of reasons a jennet may balk at motherhood including hormone imbalances, physical problems or too much human interference during that critical time when the mother and baby should be alone. Sometimes owners are too intent on making sure all goes well. They rush into the stall immediately to iodine the navel, clean soiled bedding, and help dry the foal. The bonding between the jennet and her foal takes place - or is disrupted -within the first hour following birth and the first half hour is probably the most crucial. It is during this time that the jennet smells, nuzzles and licks the foal, permanently identifying it as her own. Interference in this process by humans can disrupt the bonding. Immediately removing the placenta and drying the foal may reduce her opportunity to establish the "smell" bonding that locks the identity of her newborn into her brain.

The only truly urgent intervention needed at foaling time is if the jennet needs assistance with delivery, or if the amnion sac does not come off and the foal is unable to breath. It is crucial to iodine the navel, however this can be done is a matter of seconds.

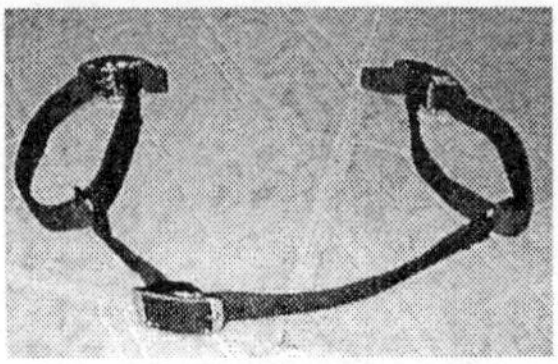

Hobbles

The first thing you should do is to tie the jennet up so that she cannot move around. If the jennet is kicking at the foal, you will need to hobble her. If you do not have a pair of equine hobbles, you can use a piece of rope or a torn T-shirt to tie her back legs together. Leave approximately 10" of space between the back legs. Be certain that you do not tie the legs too tightly and cut off her circulation! If you are using a T-shirt you need to check it every 15 minutes. Tying the back legs will enable her to walk but her attempts to kick will only amount to crow hops, not enough to actually kick and hurt her foal. You may also want to try holding up the front leg of the jennet as this can also prevent her from kicking with the back legs. You may now point the foal in the right direction of the udder. HINT: Do not grab the foal by its head and force it down to the jennet's udder. All this does is make the foal mad! Put the foal in the correct nursing position, then place one hand behind the foal - to keep it from backing up - and one hand in front of the chest of the foal - to keep it from walking forward. You may have to do this several times. Once the foal nurses, the jennet will soon associate the foal nursing with her bag becoming looser and less painful. When the foal learns where his meals are coming from, you will find that they will nurse very frequently for the first two hours. Nursing also stimulates certain hormones and the "maternal instinct".

Now let's discuss #2. The maiden jennet. Maiden jennets who attack their foals, seem to do so out of fear. They have no idea what this strange little wet thing, that caused her so much pain, is. Here at *Pheasant Meadow Farm* we have very few problems with foal rejection. I attribute this to the fact we have so many foals born here and maiden jennets are used to seeing newborns.

With maiden jennets who try to kick their foals, follow the same procedures as above. Maidens who bite their newborns need to be muzzled. If you do not have a muzzle, a temporary muzzle could be a plastic milk carton cut in half and attach it to the jennet's halter. If you have a maiden jennet biting and kicking, I would put the mother and newborn in a stall, muzzle and tie up the jennet's back legs, and leave the two of them alone for at least an hour. This means getting out of the stall and this will help with the bonding process. As soon as you see the jennet starting to accept the foal you can take the muzzle off. See how things go before untying her back legs. I have not had a jennet continue to bite the foal but have had to keep a jennet's back legs tied for up to 48 hours. Again, if you have the jennet hobbled, check to make sure they are not too tight. *NOTE: We get many calls on this subject and the "magic" hour seems to be 36 hours when a jennet decides to accept her foal so don't give up too soon.*

You generally have four hours from the time of birth until the foal starts to weaken from lack of milk. If the newborn hasn't nursed in three hours, you will have to milk the jennet to get the colostrum into the foal.

I have heard of a few occasions when people have had total rejections no matter what they do. Miniature jennet donkeys generally are wonderful mothers and I think if you try all of the above, total rejection would be even more rare.

Udder Edema in the Miniature Jennet

Occasionally, the udder and the lower abdomen become engorged with fluid due to circulatory problems. When extreme, this udder edema is sometimes confused with an umbilical hernia, a blood-filled swelling (hematoma) or an abscess. Udder edema, however, is usually characterized by an accumulation of fluid within the mammary tissue and around the lymph vessels located along the jennet's belly.

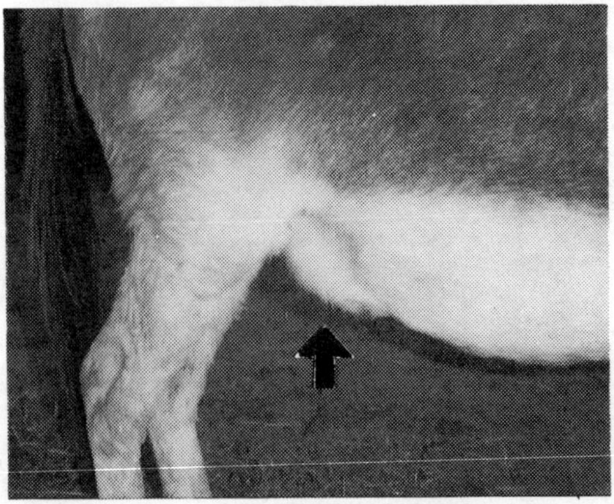

The condition, which occurs most frequently in heavy-milking jennets during early lactation and after weaning, can cause the udder to become warm and extremely painful. An emergency situation occurs when the udder is so painful that the jennet will not let her foal nurse. Severe edema predisposes the udder to infection and may prevent milk ejection.

You should call your veterinarian when you see an edema but first do a few things that your vet will surely ask about. Feel the edema, is it squashy or rock hard. Does the edema feel warm or hot to the touch? Take the jennet's temperature and report the reading to the vet.

Mild edemas will require no treatment other than exercise. Many jennets will develop a mild edema just days before she foals and it is a good indication that you can expect a baby soon. Many other jennets develop an edema within 12 to 24 hours after weaning a foal from her, and again the only treatment is exercise. It is rare, but it does happen, that a large edema will occur within two days of foaling, especially if the jennet is a heavy milk producer.

In severe cases, your veterinarian should see the jennet and he may advise massage, hand milking, cold and hot applications, and the use of mild counterirritants. He may administer diuretic drugs. Diuretics cause the shift of body waters into the urine. He may recommend lowering the jennet's salt intake in order to temporarily reduce fluid retention in body tissues. Reducing a jennet's grain intake may also help relieve swelling caused by fluid buildup within and around the mammary gland. Again, edemas are not usual]y serious, but they can become serious if you do not closely watch for changes

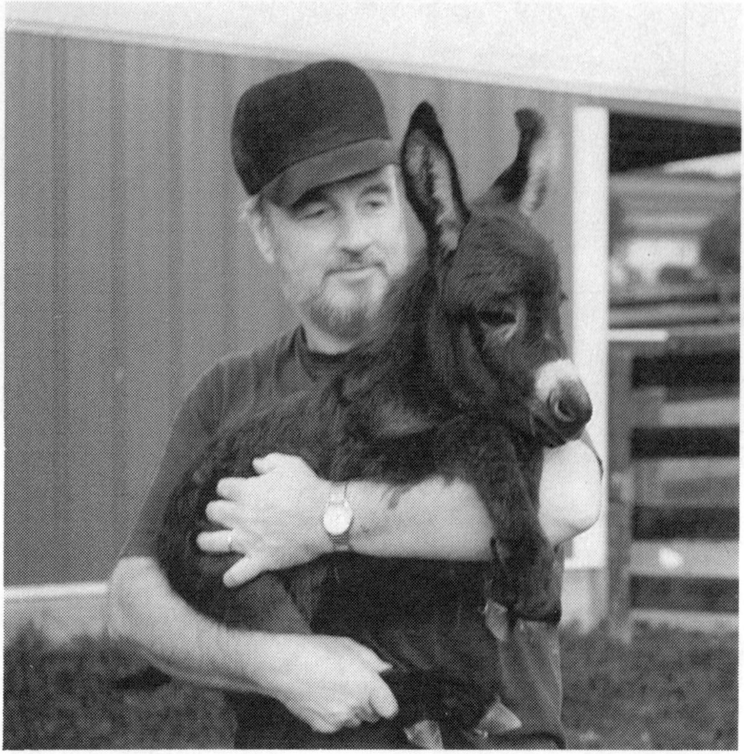

Chapter 6

The Newborn

The Importance of Colostrum

Newborn foals are susceptible to any number of infections as they are born with little or no antibodies. This is why it is so important for them to receive colostrum. Colostrum is the name given to milk produced by the jennet for the first few days after foaling. Colostrum also has a laxative effect that helps to get the newborn foal's bowels moving normally. The foal must get colostrum, if not from their mother, then from another source.

You can keep a supply of frozen colostrum in your freezer for up to 2 years. Frozen colostrum must be thawed slowly. Thawing in a pan or microwave or otherwise heating it will lead to the loss of the very antibodies that the foal needs so badly. If you want to have some colostrum on hand for emergencies, milk out a jennet who has just foaled AFTER HER FOAL has nursed six or seven times.

To prepare for the time, for whatever reason, that your foal cannot get colostrum from its mother, you should collect it from a jennet who has just foaled. The newborn or orphan who has not received any colostrum should receive two feedings of colostrum. The first feeding should be within an hour or two after birth and the second feeding a couple of hours later. Foals are only able to absorb colostrum for about 24 hours after they are born but should receive it within the first 8 hours.

Another way to get antibodies into a foal is by feeding a commercial formula available from your vet. This must be done by I.V. After 24 hours, your foal should be checked by your vet to make certain it has received adequate levels of antibodies. This is done by taking a blood test. If the test results show the foal's immunity to be low, it's too late to give additional colostrum so your vet will usually give the foal a commercially prepared serum to kick up the levels.

Sometimes donkey owners are faced with raising an orphan foal. The best solution would be a nurse jennet, however, many times nurse jennets are not available or are extremely hard to come by. Nanny goats make good foster mothers. Goats milk is higher in protein and fat but usually the difference does not cause a problem and some breeders swear by goats milk. Cow's milk MUST be altered or will cause severe diarrhea.

Passive Immunity

If the foal received adequate passive immunity via the jennet's colostrum, it is probably protected from most infectious organisms for the first three months. So at the age of 3 to 4 months, an immunization program for the foal should be started. Again, vaccinations will vary regionally. Most vets suggest an all in one vaccination containing Tetanus Toxoid, Influenza, E/W Encephalomyelitis. A separate vaccination for Rhino should also be giving - one to two weeks after the above vaccinations are given. Our experience is that giving the Rhino along with a 4 or 5 way vaccination is too much for the foal. An initial vaccination will be given at 3 to 4 months of age with a follow up booster given 30 to 50 days later.

The foal registered well above 800 milligrams/deciliter in passive transfer, but now he's going on two months of age. Just when does this immunity supplied by the mother start to taper off?

The length of time the foal will be protected from disease is largely dependent upon his dam's immunization schedule during gestation and the foal's absorption ability. If she received booster vaccinations during the last months of pregnancy, she will pass high levels of protection to her foal through her colostrum (first milk). Yet, maternal antibodies vary for different diseases. Protection against influenza, for instance, can fall off when the foal is only two months old, while encephalomyelitis immunity may last up to six months.

As often as they crop up in a herd, you would think that runny noses and occasional coughs are an unavoidable part of growing up. "The snots" afflict a youngster about the time the immunity he acquired from his dam tapers off and before his own disease-prevention system kicks in. The result is a catch all term that refers to a drippy or crusty nose, watery eyes and/or cough. A rhino vaccination greatly reduces these incidences.

Many times young donkeys between the age of five and 10 months will develop running noses for no obvious reason. Mild cases need no treatment. In fact, treating with antibiotics may interfere with the "kicking in" of the foals own immune system. Inexperienced owners may need a veterinarian to advise them whether they are in this in-between stage of a foal developing his own immunities or whether you are in fact dealing with a disease.

Developing an immunization program and keeping accurate records will benefit all the animals on your farm as well as those on your neighbors surrounding acres. And because foals are particularly susceptible to disease, care should be taken to begin vaccination before the signs of infection are obvious.

Newborn Umbilical Cord

The equine has an unusually long umbilical cord compared with other species. This provides continued communication with the mother's endometrium for up to 15 minutes after delivery. It is important to prevent premature rupture of the cord, for the intact cord provides continued maternal support to the foal. The umbilical cord contains two veins which carry the oxygen enriched blood to the foal.

The umbilical cord should remain intact until ruptured naturally. This usually occurs within 15 minutes, or less, following birth, and is caused by the foal or mothers attempts to stand. If the umbilical cord becomes severed prematurely or kinked so it restricts blood flow, the foal could be deprived of up to 1/2 pint of circulating blood. Strong pulsations of blood can be felt in the cord immediately after delivery and usually continue for one or two minutes. IF the cord breaks prematurely, do not panic as the foal will surely survive and do quite well without this extra blood.

There is a natural breaking point located about two or three inches from the foal's belly. The cord usually separates here as soon as the foal struggles. If the cord does not break naturally, grab the cord close to the foal's belly with one hand and take your other hand and place it six or seven inches down the cord and pull. You may have to pull hard. If you cannot break the cord, cut it around five inches from the foal's belly and tie it. Baling twine will work in an emergency or any other thick cord. Do not use nylon thread or fine string as that will cut through the tissue. Tie it as tightly as you can. Occasionally the placenta will come out of the jennet and all will be attached to the foal. Follow the above instructions.

Navel antiseptic should be applied as soon as the cord breaks, such as 7% tincture of iodine making sure the navel stump is well saturated before it touches any bedding or contaminants.

If you find the foal in the pasture or corral, already born and running around, it is still necessary to catch it and treat it the same way. Retreating the cord again twice within the next 48 hours gives added protection.

Trouble Signs in the Newborn

Colic In Newborns

In foals, colic within the first 48 hours of life is caused chiefly by constipation due to the retention of meconium (the foals first bowel movement). A newborns could be constipated at birth because of the hardening of the fecal mass before birth. Signs of this begin at about three hours of age where the foal will arch its back, swish its tail and stand as if it is trying to urinate. Most cases of meconium retention can be resolved by simply giving the foal a mild enema after the foal has nursed. You would use the same enema as you would for a human baby. If this does not relieve the foal, your vet should be called. NOTE: Miniature Donkeys foals do NOT ordinarily need an enema at birth as do horse foals. We at *Pheasant Meadow Farm*, after the birth of several hundred plus foals, have never had to give an enema.

Premature Breakage of the Umbilical Cord

The foal will usually lay still with occasional convulsive attacks. This is caused when the foal is deprived of a portion of its blood supply from the umbilical cord. The foal will not attempt to nurse and your vet must inject antibiotics and administer colostrum through a stomach tube.

Newborn Diarrhea (Septicemia)

A newborn with Septicemia will quickly become dehydrated with an increase in the white blood cell count. Temperatures will usually be over 102 and is caused by bacteria, viruses or fungus. It is most common in foals with a weak immune system resulting also from not receiving adequate colostrum and being born in a dirty stall. Call your vet immediately.

Any abnormal actions on the part of your foal should be reported to your vet immediately. Your foal should be bright eyed and alert from 30 minutes to three hours after birth and looking for his first meal. There is a never ending list to the problems that could develop. Your careful observation of any peculiar actions or weaknesses and prompt professional care could make the difference in whether your foal survives or not.

Is Your Newborn Really Nursing?

We get many calls from people saying "I don't think my newborn foal knows how to nurse". Some newborns are on their feet and sucking on anything in sight in a matter of minutes. Other foals may not even attempt to get up for 30 minutes and do seem to have a difficult time in understanding where their first meal is suppose to come from.

A foal needs colostrum which is filled with protective antibodies, glucose and a laxative ingredient within the first three hours of birth to get off to a good start. Many of you say the foal is in the general vicinity of the bag, but you are not sure if it is nursing.

A simple way to determine this is by feeling the jennet's udder. If it is rock hard and the teats are distended and filled with milk, then the foal is not nursing. Most foals are born with an instinctive sucking reflex. Miniature donkeys are born relatively tall compared to the height of the jennet's udder so it take a little bit of practice for the foal to understand how to lower and bend the head and neck in the right angle in order to nurse. Some foals will spend an hour sucking on the side of the stomach and leg.

To begin with, have some patience. If the foal is at least looking for the udder and the jennet is standing still and cooperating, you may want to give the foal at least 90 minutes to try and find dinner on his own. If your foal just doesn't seem to be able to get to the food source, there are some do's and don'ts here. Don't attempt to force the foal's head down to the jennet's udder and force it to nurse. All this does is make the foal concentrate on getting away from you. The proper way to help is to have someone hold the jennet still if she is moving around. Position the foal in the proper nursing position - standing along side the jennet facing toward the rear of the jennet.

Move the jennet's hind leg back so that the udder is in clear view. Follow the steps listed in **Foal Rejection** in this manner. Another little trick is to put a little milk on your finger, put it in the foal's mouth and at the same time move your finger toward the udder.

Remember, healthy foals keep the mammary gland fairly drained of milk at all times. For the first few days, examine the jennet's udder often to make sure your foal is nursing.

CPR in the Newborn Foal

Newborn foals sometimes require CPR. Therefore it is important to know how to give CPR to a foal, and to understand that it is done differently than it is in a human.

The most common cause of cardiac and/or respiratory arrest in a newborn foal is prolonged or complicated labor by the jennet. Usually the respiratory arrest occurs first. When a foal is deprived of oxygen for too long, cardiac arrest follows.

When the foal is in the jennet's uterus, it does not breathe. It gets its oxygen supply from the jennet by way of the placenta and the umbilical cord. The heart is working, of course, and has been since the foal was a tiny embryo. In a normal foaling, which is a swift procedure in equine, the separation of the foal from the jennet usually occurs when the umbilical cord ruptures, after the foal has been born. It is best to allow this to occur naturally. If the cord is cut or tied off prematurely, the foal may be deprived of a significant amount of blood from the placenta, which will ordinarily drain into the foal's body through the umbilical blood vessels. Sometimes the placenta will be delivered with the foal, although in most cases it remains behind, to drop from the jennet later. In either case, as soon as the foal loses its oxygen source - the jennet - its brain is signaled to commence breathing.

Sometimes the umbilical cord is crushed while the foal's head is still inside the jennet; or if the head has come out, it may still be in the water bag. Or perhaps the foal is coming out hind feet first. In such cases, if the umbilical source of oxygen is interrupted, the foal's brain will be signaled to start breathing. By inhaling fluids, instead of dry outside air, a foal will drown.

If the foal is not breathing, feel the chest, behind the elbow. Is there a heartbeat? If there IS a heartbeat, you do not need to do cardiac massage. Instead, start respiratory resuscitation as follows:

1. Clear the nose of fluids. These may be sucked out with a syringe, but what I usually do is pick up the foal by the hind end, and whirl it around a few times. Centrifugal force will expel fluids and mucus in the upper respiratory tract. Now, quickly begin the pulmonary resuscitation.

2. Close off one nostril. Blow into the other nostril. Unlike humans, equine cannot breathe through their mouth, so DO NOT BLOW INTO THE MOUTH.

By closing off one nostril and blowing into the other, you will effectively fill the lungs with air. A Miniature equine has lungs a little smaller than a normal size horse foal so take about 3/4's of a breath and blow into the foal's nostril while pinching off the other.

You should see the chest expand as the lungs fill with air. Then pause a moment as the lungs collapse and expel the air. Repeat this procedure, rhythmically. The rate is the same as you yourself normally breathe. If the foal starts to cough and sputter, stop for a moment to see if it has begun breathing on its own and, if so, if the breathing is strong and regular.

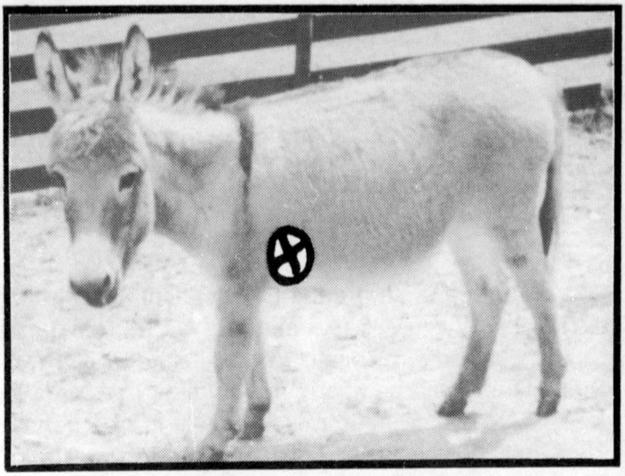

Where cardiac resuscitation is applied

If the heart has also stopped, then complete CPR if necessary. This can be done by one person, but it isn't easy. You will need to stuff something up one of the foal's nostrils to close it off while you blow in the other as already described. This will free your hands to do cardiac massage. Obviously, it is much better if one person can do the pulmonary resuscitation, while the second person does the following cardiac massage.

With the foal lying on its RIGHT side, place both hands over the lower left chest wall, just behind the foal's elbow. One hand should be on top of the other. The heel of the low hand contacts the chest wall where the heart is most superficial. With sharp but not excessive force, compress the heart and then immediately release the pressure. Repeat at one second intervals. Violent force can rupture the heart. It only takes a moderate force to compress the heart and pump blood out of it. Of course, if you feel the heartbeat start under your hand, and if it is beating regularly, stop the cardiac massage, but watch carefully in case the heart stops again.

Learning CPR may save your foal's life. It is again important to remember that when doing CPR on humans, the patient is laying on their back, while in foals they are laying on their right side.

Reference: Robert M. Miller, D.V.M. Health Problems Of The Horse

Neonatal Foal Care

Introduction

Newborn foals are vulnerable to the elements, starvation, predation, and disease. The threat of disease introduction is perhaps the greatest determinant of foal survival, with the second being exposure to risks of compromised health and injury. These hazards can be minimized through implementation of proper management practices.

Once the new foal has arrived on a bed of clean grass or fresh straw, the membranes have been cleared away, its breathing has been initiated, and it has received a vigorously stimulating rub down with a dry towel, the most critical job of observation and action begins. If the foal appears to be healthy and energetic, it is best to stand back and allow the mare and foal to bond and establish their relationship.

Delivery

The first twenty-four hours of a foal's life are the most critical. During this short time span, an alert, robust, vigorous foal can regress to irreparable states of dehydration, infection, coma, or death. A frail, lethargic foal can exhibit considerable improvement and be nearly or completely restored to stable health by the next day. Within fifteen minutes of birth, the normal foal should assume a sternal position with head upright, resting on its chest. The normal foal should stand within one hour and nurse within three hours after birth.

A healthy foal's heart rate should be greater than 60 beats per minute (bpm) at birth and increase to between 80 and 130 bpm after an hour. Within the first five days and thereafter a heart rate in the range of 80 to 120 bpm would be considered normal. A heart murmur may be heard a birth, but should be gone before the fourth day. The foal should be breathing at a rate of 60 to 80 breaths per minute at birth, and the rate should then decrease to between 30 and 40 breaths per minute after an hour. The normal foal's temperature should be in the range of 99 to 102 degrees. After the foal has become somewhat acclimated to life outside the womb, it should stand, nurse, and move around the stall showing normal inquisitive activity. The normal foal lies down to rest frequently for short naps throughout the day.

Immunity

Intrauterine antibodies are not provided to the foal by the mare during gestation. Antibodies are too large to pass through the mare's thick placenta and into the foal's bloodstream. The immunity that is provided is available only through the antibodies in her first milk, the colostrum. The colostrum, however, is available for only forty-eight hours after which it is replaced by normal milk, which has no immunity value. Ingestion of colostrum is therefore the most critical factor influencing the foal's survival, growth, and future potential.

The foal's ability to absorb antibodies through the lining of the duodenum is based on the presence of special absorption cells in the small intestine. These special cells decrease rapidly over the first twenty-four hours; after forty-eight hours they are replaced with normal duodenal lining. Thus, a foal can only absorb antibodies during the first two days; it absorbs most of the antibodies within its first eight hours of life. For this reason, it is extremely important that the foal receive colostrum during the first eight hours of life to receive the antibodies it will need for immunity in the following three to four months.

The process by which antibodies are passed from mare to foal is called passive transfer. Occasionally a foal exhibits a failure of passive transfer where, even though the antibodies are readily available in the colostrum, the foal is unable to absorb and use them. An immunoglobulin, IgG, test can be performed to identify failure of passive transfer of blood. An immunoglobulin level of less than 600-800 mg/dl indicates a problem. Blood IgG levels below 400 mg/dl indicates a failure of passive transfer, and a veterinarian should be consulted.

Antibodies against certain diseases will be present in the mare's colostrum if she is vaccinated with booster injections thirty days prior to parturition. Tetanus is one disease to which equine are extremely susceptible. The mare should be vaccinated against all common diseases, because the colostrum can only contain antibodies against diseases to which the mare has been exposed. If the mare has not been given a tetanus toxoid thirty days prior to parturition, then the foal should be given 1500 IU of tetanus antitoxin at birth in order to protect it from the tetanus pathogen which is ever present in equine feces. No antibiotics or probiotics, such as special vitamin formulations, should be administered the first day of life in an effort to bolster the foal's vigor. These tend only to increase perinatal morbidity and diarrhea.

In the case of an aglactic mare (one that does not produce milk in adequate quantities), a mare with poor-quality colostrum, one that leaked her colostrum, or one that is dead, a source of frozen colostrum taken from other mares will provide the foal with the immune protection it needs.

Milking 6 to 8 ounces of colostrum from all mares after their foals have suckled will provide a reserve which can be frozen. It is a good idea to have this resource on hand even if no problems are expected. When used, this colostrum should be slowly heated, not microwaved, to body temperature. Microwaving destroys the protein molecules that make the antibodies protective. The best colostrum sources will be from mares on the same farm as the foal in order to provide the most specific immunity. Nurse mares can be used as a source of milk.

Premature Foals

Foals that arrive prematurely will be especially susceptible to risks of the environment and disease. Since their bodies are physiologically underdeveloped, they are unprepared, even with sufficient colostrum, to provide adequate resistance to disease. The lungs of premature foals are especially underdeveloped. They tend to have low body temperatures, are especially susceptible to colds, infections, hypothermia, and require a lot of intensive care to survive.

Neonatal Procedures

After the foal's birth, the first important task is treatment of the foal's navel with a tincture of iodine solution. The umbilical cord should be allowed to sever naturally, rather than cutting or tying it off. The navel stump should then be saturated with tincture of iodine immediately after tearing. The importance of this simple task can not be overstated. Treating the navel stump will prevent joint infection or Navel Ill. This is a bacterial infection usually resulting from poor navel treatment and umbilical infection as its source. It develops in foals less than thirty days of age and is considered a medical emergency. Aggressive therapy is needed to prevent permanent cartilage or bone damage. Symptoms of joint ill include sudden lameness with or without systemic illness, swollen and painful joints, and stiffness. More than one joint may be involved, such as stiffness through the back or neck pain.

The navel stump is an ideal growth environment and entrance for potentially life threatening bacteria into the system of the newborn. A simple iodine treatment minimizes the risks of navel ill and other infections quickly and easily. The treatment should be repeated daily until the navel stump is completely dry. Continue to examine the navel daily until it becomes dry, shrinks, and disappears altogether. If the navel does not close properly, or begins to leak urine, there may be a need for additional treatment and veterinary attention.

Although I have never once had to give a donkey foal an enema, on rare occasions they are needed. An enema is used to treat and prevent meconium retention. The foal's rectum and anus are easily damaged. The enema should be administered with one pint of warm, soapy water through a soft, narrow, pliable rubber tube inserted no more than four to five inches into the rectum. Mixtures of warm water and mineral oil or commercially obtained human FLEET enemas can also be used. Remember, during the first part of the foal's life, infection and disease are constant threats. The stall and bedding should be frequently cleaned and conditions kept as sanitary as possible. Exercise often helps foals pass their meconium. Weather permitting, a foal with signs of impaction should be turned out.

Scouting for Problems

When observing your foal, you can use as a check list to scout for problems and catch them as soon as they get started. Remember, foals can go from apparent health to extreme illness in less than 24 hours.

* A normal foal eats, sleeps, rests, defecates, and urinates in short, constant cycles. It should never do one for an excessively long period of time or stop doing one altogether.

* The normal foal is curious, alert, and aware of surroundings, using all of its available senses. The first area to watch is the nursing habits. A healthy foal will keep the dam's udder drained at all times. Decreased consumption indicated by a build up of milk in the udder and drops accumulating on the teats are a sign of a problem. When intake is decreased, degeneration in the condition of the foal is shockingly disproportionate. Depression, weakness, and evidence of residual milk on the foal's face ("milky nose") are signs of a weak foal. If these signs are observed, take the foal's temperature immediately. A reading higher or lower than the normal 99 to 102 degree range by more than two tenths of a degree warrants concern. If the foal is nursing constantly, the mare may not be producing enough milk and the foal may be malnourished.

* Most foals initially have a fear of humans, thus any foal that you can walk up to, catch, and easily handle should be examined further.

* A normal foal takes short, frequent naps. The disturbed foal should be immediately alert, getting to its feet and moving around. When resting, the respiration rate should be an even 30 to 40 breaths per minute.

* A normal foal urinates and defecates frequently in small amounts. Urination should occur without straining in an even flow. A foal commonly urinates immediately after standing up from a nap. With colts, be sure that

the penis extends beyond the prepuce during urination. If retracted, this will cause irritation and prevent the navel from drying properly. It is not uncommon for the penis to be extended much of the time in colts less than 18 months of age.

* A foal that is having trouble defecating will stand and strain, with tail elevated to no avail. It may walk around stiffly with tail elevated and may stretch in an attempt to alleviate the discomfort or pain. A foal with acute constipation will roll over on its back and stretch its legs out in a characteristic position, with neck extended back and knees pulled up toward the head as far as possible.

* The foal's immediate environment should be carefully scrutinized for hazards, obstructions, openings that the foal could become wedged or caught in (they can do so in extremely small areas), and protrusions. Bear in mind that a foal may move while lying down or roll underneath a fence or manger and become trapped. The temperature should be kept moderate and comfortable for the first twenty-four hours. An adequate supply of straw bedding in the stall will provide more than enough trapped, warm air to keep the foal from becoming chilled. As long as the area is well-ventilated and dry, the temperature after twenty-four hours postpartum is not a major concern. Many respiratory problems are caused by mare and foal housing areas being heated and poorly ventilated. Mares and foals do much better in unheated, well-ventilated stalls free of direct drafts, or, better yet, when outdoors.

Turn-out/Exercise

The timing for a mare and foal to be first turned out depends on the climate, time of year of foaling, and weather conditions. Turn-out on the first day after birth is fine if the temperature is mild and it is not icy or muddy. The pair should not be allowed to become fatigued or overly stressed by temperature extremes or by overheating as a result of exercise or excitement.

Observation will be required for the following ten days, as problems could still occur. The mare's udder should be closely watched and the foal's temperature monitored daily. A subnormal, out of range, temperature indicates an infection and requires immediate attention.

Pediatric Problems

Pediatric problems may be divided into three categories: prenatal (before birth), perinatal (during birth), and neonatal (after birth to two weeks of age). This publication is primarily concerned with the neonatal pediatric problems.

Septicemia (bacterial blood infection) may develop in utero and be present at birth or onset around three days of age. Bacterial infections are responsible for one-third of all foal mortality occurring within the first two months of age. Once a foal becomes sick, it needs immediate veterinary treatment and care. Infections are aggravated by prematurity, delayed or inadequate quantity of colostrum, or anything that diminishes the quality of the foal's immune response. A septicemic foal will appear sleepy: depressed, lethargic, and may exhibit decreased suckling, dehydration, hypothermia, fever, diarrhea, or respiratory distress.

Septicemic infections may be prevented by maintaining good mare health, a clean environment, administering proper umbilical care and disinfection, and ensuring prompt ingestion of adequate amounts of colostrum. Although not a cause for septicemia, administering tetanus toxoid to the mare three weeks prior to delivery or 1500 IU of antitoxin to the foal at birth will protect against tetanus, which is one of the most serious bacterial infections for both adult and newborn horses.

Viremia (viral infection) may present itself in a wide variety of ways. Listed here are several common viruses:

* Congenital Equine Herpes-1, produces a weak, immune-deficient foal. Invariably fatal.

* Rotavirus causes debilitating diarrhea.

* Coronavirus causes severe diarrhea.

Botulism or "Shaker Foal", is caused by the botulism bacteria and may have a rapid (12-36 hour) or gradual (2-4 day) onset. It is most common in foals less than eight weeks old, but may occur up to eight months of age. Shaker foal syndrome is characterized by an inability to swallow, slow responses, dilated pupils, and muscle weakness. It may be treated with botulism antitoxin and penicillin.

Pneumonia is commonly seen as a secondary development to bacterial or viral infection. Scout for pneumonia by looking for increases in the foal's resting respiration rate. The foal may have a runny nose, depressed and unthrifty look, be unwilling to nurse, and may cough. Temperature should be taken on a suspected case of pneumonia as temperature will usually be elevated. Any increase in temperature or respiration not explained by ambient temperature or exercise should receive immediate attention.

Pneumonia in foals, and equine in general, is complicated by the lack of significant coughing as a symptom and defense mechanism. Often, a case of pneumonia may appear completely normal without obvious abnormal signs until the condition is so advanced that aggressive treatment is needed. Premature and dysmature foals are most susceptible to pneumonia.

Diarrhea, most commonly of nutritional, viral, or bacterial origin in foals, can be initiated by sudden diet change, over consumption of milk, ingestion of foreign material, parasites, carbohydrate intolerance, and water intake while nursing. Foals will usually show signs of diarrhea during the mare's foal heat about 6-10 days postpartum. This diarrhea is normal and does not harm the foal in any way. At this time the foal's gastrointestinal tract is undergoing physiologic alteration, and the microflora that inhabit the tract and contribute to its normal functioning are adapting to the digestion of solid foods. Most foals will improve if simply left alone.

The parasites responsible for foal diarrhea are Strongyloides (threadworms) and ascarids (lung worms). These can be prevented by a good deworming program for the mare and foal. The primary viral source of foal diarrhea is rotavirus which often occurs as an epidemic in foals less than two months old. The source of this virus may be adults that shed the virus into their environment, yet themselves don't have diarrhea. Some farms seem to have problems because of the large number of virus in their environment.

Salmonella bacteria are the most dangerous cause of bacterial diarrhea. A bloody hemorrhagic diarrhea especially is indicative of Salmonella. The source of salmonella infection is carrier horses that shed the bacteria into the environment. Antibiotic, fluid, and electrolyte therapies are effective against this type of bacteria.

Ruptured bladder is rare, but when present, occurs ninety percent of the time in colts between one and two days of age. This condition requires corrective surgery. Its telltale symptoms include: depression, gradual loss of appetite, abdominal distension (with or without abdominal pain), and decreased frequency and volume of urine. If not corrected surgically, coma or death will occur. A foal with a ruptured bladder may flex its back and extend its legs out in front and behind and may resemble a constipated foal. Because of these symptoms, a veterinarian should be consulted if straining is not relieved by an enema.

Patent urachus, most common in male foals, refers to urine leaking from the navel. This condition arises usually within the first two weeks from an incomplete closure of the urachus, the tube which connects the bladder to the ubillicus in the fetal foal. Urine may leak into the abdominal cavity or surrounding subcutaneous tissues should the urachus be open between the umbilicus and bladder. Treatment for patent urachus may be either medical or surgical. Foals with other infections may develop a patent urachus secondarily. Surgery is generally required for foals that develop infection associated with a patent urachus. If the urachus is not infected, it may close on its own in two days or may be medicated until it closes.

Navel problems generally occur in one of two forms, abscesses or hernias. A navel abscess occurs sometime after the foal is one week old and may or may not be associated with signs of systemic infection. An abscessed navel will appear enlarged and may be hot, swollen, or painful. Hernias usually occur at birth, but go unnoticed until weeks later. The size of the opening in the abdominal wall determines what form of treatment is necessary. If larger then two fingers in diameter (2 to 3 inches), the intestines may become trapped and surgery is recommended.

Neonatal Maladjustment Syndrome (NMS) is a term used to describe neurologic problems which develop within 72 hours of birth and are characterized by an inability to stand, disorientation and struggling, loss of affinity for the mare and nursing, a poor sucking reflex, blindness or convulsions, and a characteristic airway-origin barking noise, hence the nick-name "barker foals." A Barker or NMS foal may or may not be the result of an abnormal birth. Causes may be the result of a decreased oxygen supply to the foal associated with traumatic or prolonged birth, in-utero infection, or central nervous system hemorrhage or swelling, but it is not infectious. The survival rate related with this disorder is 50 percent; it is almost always hopeless if there is no improvement within six days of onset.

A premature or weak foal requires special assistance and considerations. Length of gestation alone is a poor indicator of the individual foal's readiness for birth and maturity. In-utero growth retardation can occur as a result of several conditions including in-utero infection, multiple pregnancy, malnutrition, and infection of the placenta.

A premature foal is weaker and will take a longer time to rise after birth. It will usually exhibit a depressed sucking ability, decreased birth weight, and may have a more dome-shaped head or floppy ears and red tongue. Difficult breathing, increased respiration rate, and reduced body temperature coupled with susceptibility to hypothermia are characteristics associated with prematurity. They often have weak flexor tendons and suspensory ligaments and walk on their fetlocks rather than their hooves at birth. These foals require special assistance and support through environmental temperature regulation and augmented nutrition. Special consideration needs to be given to prevention and control of infection where such a disease susceptible foal is concerned. Respiratory support with oxygen may also be needed in case of incompletely developed lungs.

Gastric ulcers occur when the protective factors of the stomach lining cells are disturbed. This causes a breakdown of mucous and cell membrane barriers which protect stomach cells from acid damage. Foals with ulcers show signs of colic, grind their teeth, and salivate excessively. Several causes of ulcers have been suggested including bacteria, viruses, stress, foreign material in the digestive tract, and some drugs. Treat ulcers with antacids to neutralize the acidity of the intestine and with other medications to protect the damaged ulcer site, inhibit acid production, and promote stomach-wall healing.

Lateral leg deformities can appear severe at birth and make profound improvements within a few days. Usually this is a result of positioning in the uterus and poor tendon tone from not being used. Most legs straighten in the first week of life with no treatment. If legs are not improving in angle of pasterns, direction of hooves and straightness of knees and bones, splinting may be needed. Experienced assistance will determine whether exercise, splinting (with lots of padding), or surgery is needed. The younger these cases receive veterinary attention, the greater will be their success. When the foal is first born, the sole of the foot will be covered with extensions of soft hoof tissue called "feathers" that protected the mare's reproductive tract from damage by the sharp hooves during birth. These feathers dry up and disappear quite naturally on their own if left alone.

The growth rate of foals' hooves varies greatly from one foal to the next, but foals of this young age require very little attention to their hooves, other than an occasional rasping-off of toes that become too pointed. This trimming prevents the hoof from "breaking over" to the sides and causing stress on leg joints and tendons. If the legs are crooked, some corrective trimming in the first four weeks of age may is beneficial.

Care Through Four Weeks

A foal gains weight very rapidly during the first month and weight gain is directly proportional to the daily energy consumption. Optimum levels are not known with certainty, but a gain of 2 percent of body weight per day is healthy. Some references suggest 3 to 3.25 percent; however, this may promote bone growth problems. A creep feed should contain 15% crude protein, .6% lysine, .7% calcium, and .4% phosphorus, calculated as percents of the total ration. A chopped hay and grain mixture can be fed free choice, but straight grain rations should be limit fed. This feeding system can be continued to augment mare's milk until the foal is weaned, usually at four months of age.

Conclusion

A new foal represents many possibilities to its owners: the beginning of a new training prospect, a future stakes winner, a continuation of superior performance bloodlines, new stock to augment a breeding program, or a fine, dependable work and pleasure animal.

The achievements that the foal embodies will happen only if the foal is given every opportunity to grow and develop to the fullest of its genetic potential. Allowing this potential to be expressed comes through careful attention to detail and continual observation. The earlier a problem is detected, the easier it is to resolve the situation. The nutrition, health care, and time invested in observing and handling this foal are only the beginning of his progress. Judicious, educated management needs to be a continuing process throughout the formative years and beyond if champions are to be produced.

Reference: Cooperative Extension Service, Purdue University Brenda Weedman, Department of Animal Sciences; Janice Sojka, VMD, Veterinary Clinical Sciences; and Mark Russell, PhD, Department of Animal Sciences

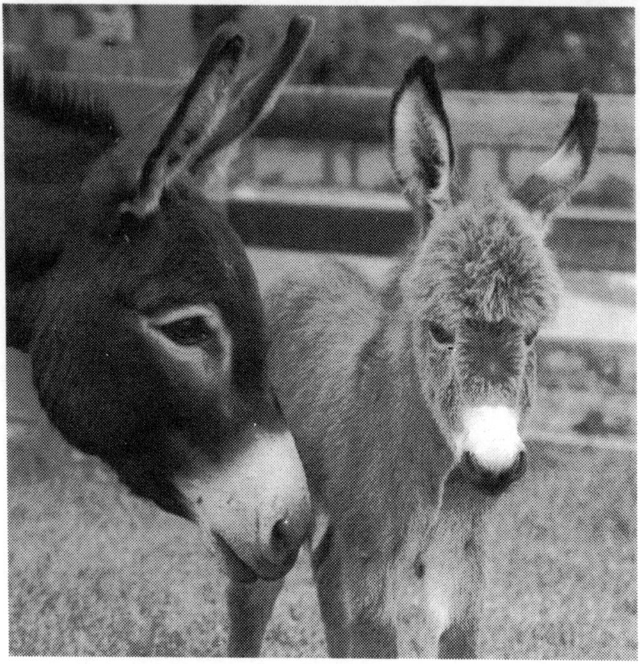

When A Little Extra Help is Needed

How to give a sick foal a fighting chance

Sometimes things go wrong. The foal that a few hours ago looked fine is now lethargic, standing with head down and ignoring his dam. The foal that should have arrived in perfect health instead lies prone and is not adjusting to life outside the uterus.

What can you do when faced with an ill foal? Although any number of pathogens, accidents or internal factors could have induced the youngsters problem, you first and most important step is to arrange veterinary evaluation and treatment *immediately.*

If you and your veterinarian agree that a trip to your regional neonatal intensive-care clinic is warranted, then it is absolutely necessary to alert the clinic that a foal is on the way. Inform the clinicians of your "ETA" - estimated time of arrival. The stall will need time to prepare, and an advance call could save your foal's life.

Don't "Wait and See"

According to Elizabeth Morris, DVS, a researcher at Tufts University neonatal foal unit in Massachusetts, there is a direct correlation between the speed with which a sick foal received treatment and the prognosis for his recovery. This may mean putting the young foal in the station wagon or utility vehicle and bring the mare/jennet later.

Even if the nearest equine hospital is only 20 minutes away, delaying treatment while making arrangements to transport the mare/jennet could compromise the neonate's condition. However, bring his dam along as soon as possible - within a few hours. The mare/jennet may not accept the foal if they are reunited after much time has elapsed.

Once the foal is headed for the clinic, there is a lot you can do to keep his condition from deteriorating during the trip. According to Morris, your top priority is to keep him warm. Prop the foal in an upright (sternal) position and keep him sung with blankets. Have someone sit next to him to provide additional warmth and support and to prevent him from flailing.

Your next goal is to prevent dehydration and malnourishment. A foal becomes critically dehydrated about six hours after ceasing to nurse (and could be sooner for miniatures). If he is also suffering from diarrhea, he will become dehydrated much faster. In addition, his bloodstream is rapidly depleted of energy and protein once nursing stops.

If the foal will suckle, feed him milk replacer (or goats milk is even better) through a bottle until he can be reunited with his dam. During foaling season you should have on hand a package or two of high-quality milk replacer - a product with easily digestible carbohydrates and a good protein source (again, goat's milk is also well accepted by sick foals.)

High quality milk replacers are well worth the investment. Research at the University of California-Davis has shown that, compared to healthy neonates, sick foal have changes in their blood-protein concentrations consistent with malnutrition. Sick human babies have been shown to do much better when fed a protein supplement. The sicker the foal, the less he will tolerate being fed, and very ill youngsters may not be able to digest certain ingredients in lower-quality milk replacers.

At The Clinic: Speeders Treatment

Keeping him warm, keeping him fed and supporting his immune system may be the difference between a foal who is sick but can survive a trip to the clinic and a foal that arrives in shock and near death. Yet, there is more you can do to assist in treatment once the foal is in the hands of a veterinarian.

Be ready with the foal's history. The clinicians will need it to initiate appropriate treatment and arrive at an accurate diagnosis.

Reference: Written by Leslie Kelly

What's Wrong With My Foal

Sponsored by Mare's Match Foal Mill Replacer from Land O' Lakes

How bad is it Doc?

G - Generally not life-threatening; treat & watch for complications

V - Variable: foals usually respond to prompt treatment

N - Not life-threatening, but not curable

R - Red Alert: Life threatening

M - Most often fatal

What You See	Looking Closer		Probable Diagnosis	What Can Be Done
Breathing labored, suppressed or noisy	Soreness, reluctance to move	G	Broken ribs due to severe compression during delivery	Stall rest, gentle handing
	Reluctance to move or nurse, extended abdomen, "sawhorse" stance	M	Ruptured diaphragm, often due to birth trauma	Immediate corrective surgery, prognosis grave
	Yellowish-stained amniotic fluid with delivery	R	Meconium-aspiration pneumonia	Antibiotics
	Depression, coughing, intermittent fever beginning at 2 weeks to 3 months	R	Foal pneumonia	Specific antibiotics, based on ID of bacteria from direct sample - R equi a common culprit
	Cough, debility, progressive illness in spit of treatment	M	Combined immunodeficiency; genetic lack of immune system	Always fatal, by 3-6 months
Deformity	Leg joints misaligned - bowlegged or knock-kneed	V	Angular limb deformity	Brace; surgery; stall rest
	Tight-shortened tendons, forced foal to knuckle-forward	R	Contracted tendons, congenital or acquired	Surgery for moderate cases, euthanasia for severe
	Fetlocks on ground	G	Ligament-tendon laxity	Rest, intermittent bracing
	Overshot or undershot jaw	G	Jaw deformity	If not overly severe, it generally corrects itself in 3 months

What You See	Looking Closer		Probable Diagnosis	What Can Be Done
Deformity - con't	Extra toes or other parts	V	Developmental error	Surgical Removal
	Legs bent up, stiff, twisted, foal possibly undeliverable without surgery	M	Contracted foal	Foal usually born dead; euthanize
	Enlarged head, Hunchback, or other severe deformity	M	Congenital, nongenetic defect	Survival, usefulness unlikely
Weakness, Incoordination Muscle weakness Sudden loss of vigor	Delivery between 325-350 days, soft haircoat, floppy ears, low birthweight, little or no suckle strength, week fetlocks	R	Prematurity or dysmaturity if delivery occurred at or near term	Oxygen, humidity and temperature control, tube feeding, fluids
	Intolerance of exercise	V	Congenital heart defect	Cardovascular exam, possibly surgery
	Will not nurse, severe diarrhea dehydration, subnormal temp bluish-white third eyelid	R	"Sleeper foal", caused by Actinobacillus bacteria	Antibiotics, fluids, prognosis poor
	Inflammation of umbilical vein, fever, depression	R	Navel Ill - Septicemia; systemic bacterial infection of bloodstream	Specific antibiotics,fluids, intensive nursing care, in newborn administer plasma
Sudden loss of vigor with 12-36 hours of 1st nursing	Urine shaded pink or red, if condition persists, oral membranes and eye whites turn yellow	R	Neonatal isoerythrolysis, also know as yellow foal or hemolytic icterus; due to incompatible blood types of mother & foal	Confirm with jaundiced foal agglutination test, stop foal from nursing if diagnosed within 24 hours of birth, milk out mothers colostrum, bottle feed foal until after 36 hours old
Jennet cannot nurse foal	Jennet dies, does not allow nursing or is unable to provide milk	R	Orphan or rejected foal; agalactic mare; early weaning	Supply colostrum to newborn provide ongoing nourishment with foal milk replacer or obtain a nurse goat. (goats milk would be first choice. for donkeys)

What You See	Looking Closer		Probable Diagnosis	What Can Be Done
Straining	Tall switching, meconium not passed	V	Simple constipation	Enema, fluids
	Distended abdomen, little or no urine produced, jaundiced membranes, fever, progressive weakness	R	Ruptured bladder due to birth trauma or jerk on umbilical cord after delivery	Surgery to repair bladder, drain urine from abdomen, fluids
Bulge under skin	Fluid-like oval bubble in umbilical region, easily pushed back inside	G	Umbilical hernia due to compression during delivery or other trauma	Most spontaneously close, few need external support or surgically corrected
	Bulge of organ/tissue in scrotal area	G	Scrotal hernia	Surgical repair
	Progressive enlargement behind jaw, may resonate when tapped	V	Tympany of the gutteral pouch	Surgery of faulty pouch opening
	Bulge in front of ear	V	Dentigerous cyst	Surgery to remove anomalous tooth
Low Immunoglobulin Count	Less than 400 mg	R	Failure of passive transfer, foal did not receive adequate immunity from colostrum	Administer fresh/frozen colostrum if dam's colostrum is deficient and foal is less than 24 hrs old; otherwise plasma transfusion
	Greater than 400 mg low risk environment	G	Partial failure of passive transfer	Foal probably adequately protected
	Less than 800 mg high risk environment	R	Failure of passive transfer	Administer plasma, continue monitoring Ig level
Loose Stools	Mild diarrhea coinciding w/dam's foal heat, foal remains alert	G	Transient, 9-day scours	Gently clean foal's tall & buttock area and apply Vaseline

What You See	Looking Closer		Probable Diagnosis	What Can Be Done
	Dehydration, scalding of skin on buttocks, matting of tail	V	Noninfectious diarrhea, due to over-eating too rich milk, eating manure, etc	Fluids, decreased-diluted rations, clean tail as above give 5 cc's Kaopectate
	Rapid dehydration, scalding, matting, fever, depression	R	Infectious diarrhea	Antibiotics, fluids, clean tail and buttocks, Kaopectate
Colicky	Colicky after ingesting first milk, enema ineffective	R	Closed colon or rectum, developmental error	Surgery
	Rolling, thrashing, lying on back, fecal matter no passed	R	Severe constipation, fecal mass too large or too far forward for enema	Mineral oil, milk of magnesia, caster oil, fluids, sedation
	Lethargy, loss of appetite, diarrhea, teeth grinding, lying on back	V	Ulcer	Confirm with endoscopy, treat
Profuse watery discharge at eyes	Blinking, avoidance of light scratched cornea	G	Inversion of eyelid, dehydration	Fluids, lubricate eye
Navel Stump dripping urine	Wet, soiled, warm, swollen navel stump	V	Failure of umbilical stump to close	Daily cauterization with double strength tincture of iodine
Swollen Joints	Joints hot, painful, lameness, fever, depression	R	Joint-Ill - bone infection	Specific antibiotics, surgical draining, prognosis poor
Incoordination - Muscle weakness	Head & body tremors, progressively interfering w/normal depression	M	Genetic incompletion	No known treatment
	Loss of appetite, progressive muscle weakness, muscle tremors causing knee quiver	R	Shaker-foal syndrome	Treat w/antitoxin, muscle stimulants, calcium injection, penicillin fluids
	Sudden loss of muscle tone, fainting, sudden sleeping spells	G	Narcolepsy - neurological sleep attacks	Usually self-correcting within 1-2 weeks

Premature Foals

Premature foals in horses are fairly easy to determine as they have a well defined length of pregnancy. It is more difficult with miniature donkey foals as they are known to carry a foal from 11 months, 1 week to in excess of 13 months. The average gestation for a miniature donkey is 11 months, 3 weeks, 4 days.

Certain characteristics go along with prematurity such as general weakness, low birth weight, reduced sucking reflex, delay in standing and inability to maintain body temperature. The first three days are critical. During this time, some foals die due to general collapse of neurological and cardiopulmonary functions.

"Bambi" was scheduled to be put in the foaling stall the next evening for night time observation by our barn to house TV monitors. Instead, she decided to go down to the woods sometime around midnight and have her foal in the muddiest place she could find next to our stream. We discovered the foal the next morning, covered in mud and very weak. The foal was wobbly on her feet, head hung low and ears laid back. Immediately after calling the vet, we felt Bambi's udder and deducted that the foal had not yet nursed. We milked her and force fed the foal 1/4 cup of colostrum, over a period of several hours with a syringe as she had no noticeable sucking reflex. Her foal, "Pixie", was given a tetanus antitoxin vaccination. Although the air temp was around 65 degrees, we knew Pixie could not regulate her own body temperature, so we turned on the heat in the foaling stall. Within two hours she started to perk up yet still had no sucking reflex. When the vet arrived, we held the foal up to the mother's udder and milked her - squirting the milk into Pixie's mouth. Because of her tiny size, the vet did not want to pass a stomach tube unless absolutely necessary. Within several hours, Pixie was nursing on her own.

Pixie's teeth did not start to break through her gums until around day 15 whereas a full term foal starts at 4 or 5 days. Mentally, we feel she was normal from day one. She was physically much weaker than a full term foal and for the first week, tired very easily.

How you can tell you have a Premature Foal

The term premature can be difficult to determine as it applies to the gestation of a Miniature Donkey jennets. Jennets are individuals and have been known to carry a foal anywhere from 11 to 13 months therefore, determining prematurely can be very difficult. Generally, a foal born before a gestation of 11 months, 1 week would be termed premature, although some jennets routinely deliver a full term foal at 11 months, year after year. Weather conditions can be very influential as to when a jennet will deliver. Here on the east coast, and especially in the winter, we have found a definite correlation between a rise in humidity which usually means rain and/or warmer temperatures.

Characteristics of Premature Foals:

General weakness
Low birth weight
Reduced sucking reflex
Delay in standing
Inability to maintain body temperature
Ears flopped downward and backward
Difficulty in establishing a normal jennet/foal relationship.

The tongue of the premature foal is often deep red, and the skin is usually very silky. A premature foal is at a disadvantage as it departs the intrauterine protection well before it has received full nourishment or fully developed faculties required for survival. Premature foals can develop normal behavior patterns within a week, but the first three days are very critical. During this time, some foals die due to general collapse of neurological and cardiopulmonary functions.

Since equine fetal growth is greatly intensified during the last two months of gestation, any reduction of this growth period lessens the chances of survival. Some people consider any foal born two weeks "early" as a "preemie". I have seen "early" foals born so strong and vigorous and healthy that without the records and dates, no one could prove that they were truly premature. It has, however, been agreed upon that any foal arriving before 11 months gestation has little chance for survival, if it is born alive.

Premature foals are primarily noted for poor lung-tissue expansion and reduced oxygenation, nonfunctional gastrointestinal tracts and subnormal temperatures. An incubator can help with all of these problems.

Care of the premature foal includes maintaining the foal in the most supportive environment possible. The best environment is achieved through the use of an incubator, which allows the temperature, oxygen content, and humidity of the foal's surroundings to be controlled.

Incubators are expensive and not all veterinarian clinics have them. If one is not available, a well bedded stall with several heat lamps will work. The importance of elevating and establishing the body temperature cannot be overemphasized. The foal should be fed its mother's milk through a tube or by means of a bottle every one or two hours until it is able to rise and nurse on its own. Most importantly, the jennet's colostrum should be milked and given to the foal as soon as possible, preferably within 3 hours of birth. Do not feed any other type of milk replacer or goats milk until you have fed the colostrum.

Encourage the foal to stand while you support it. This will help strengthen its muscles. If you can bottle feed the foal, have a helper hold the foal up. The longer it lies and is fed, the more it will adopt a helpless, passive attitude. Be sure to keep the jennet milked out until the foal is able to nurse on a regular basis.

Testing for Antibodies in the Newborn

As of a few years ago, no one that we know of had ever tested the newborn donkey foal for antibodies. Our vets did not know for certain if the test would even work on donkeys so we had a newborn tested and found that the test is reliable for donkeys.

Blood is taken from the foal between 24 and 48 hours of age. The blood serum is tested against specific antigens (foreign compounds that stimulate the production of antibodies) to determine the concentration of antibodies in the serum. Your vet can either send the blood serum to a lab for analysis, which is quite expensive, however gives very accurate counts, or they can test the blood in their own clinics which will give you somewhat sufficient counts.

The test kits that your vet uses gives only three different results. 400 plus indicates that the foal has plenty of antibodies in its blood. 200 to 400 indicates passive or adequate antibodies. Less than 200 indicates failure of passive transfer - none or very little antibodies were received and/or utilized by the foal. "Failure of Passive Transfer" may occur when the jennet drips milk for several hours or days prior to giving birth or a foal who does not nurse within the first 3 or 4 hours of birth. Some horse breeders routinely have their foals checked.

Foal Diarrhea

It can be deadly to a Miniature

Diarrhea in foals (also called scours) is frequently due to bacterial infection, although some diarrhea in foals in probably caused by viruses. The animal is generally weaken by other factors. He may have been weak and chilled by bad weather right after he was born. He may have been born in a dirty environment and picked up infection in a contaminated stall. Diarrhea in foals also may be seen with a jennet who is a good milker and a foal who is greedy and actually getting more than his body can actually digest.

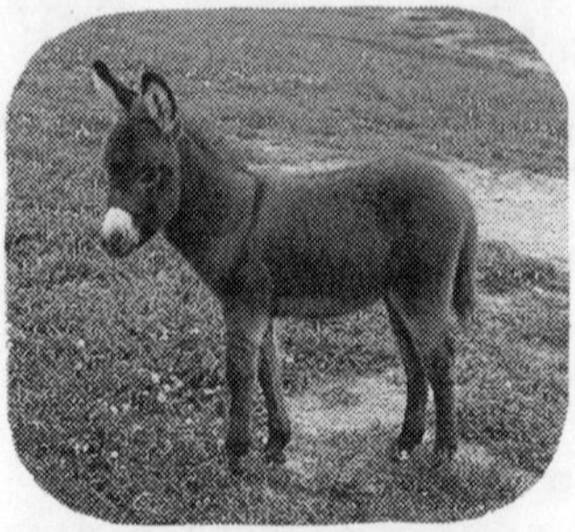

According to Roberta Dwyer, DVM, Diplomat American College of Veterinary Preventative Medicine, of the Gluck Equine Research Center in Lexington, many factors play into the equation of whether a foal will be afflicted with diarrhea. The main factor usually is associated with whether the foal received enough maternal colostrum, and if the colostrum contained enough antibodies to ward off the viruses and bacteria that the new foal faces in the first few weeks of life.

The causative agents for diarrhea can be bacteria viruses, or a range of non-infectious agents or conditions such as toxins, lactose intolerance, or "foal heat" diarrhea. Infectious agents that can cause diarrhea include rotavirus, Actinobacillus, Rhodoccus equi, clostridial organisms, and Salmonella. One must remember that when it comes to diarrhea, it is often hard to diagnose the specific cause.

"Only 50% of individual cases of diarrhea are ever documented after testing to be caused by a specific agent," Dwyer said. "This is the same with people; 50% of the patients in hospitals who come in with diarrhea are never diagnosed. They're put through a battery of tests, and it can still remain unknown whether it was toxic, infectious, or if they ate ten pounds of peanut M&Ms."

The foal may show scours when the jennet comes into heat. This is called 'foal heat diarrhea.' It was once thought that this was due to hormonal changes appearing in the jennet and therefore in her milk, however it is also seen in orphan foals being fed milk replacer. This typical diarrhea which first appears at 7-9 days, is now thought to come from bacteria entering the foal's digestive system for the first time. Foal heat diarrhea, although something you should keep an eye on especially in miniatures, generally does not show complications and there should be no temperature rise. Reducing the amount of grain given to jennets who are nursing foals at this time may help reduce the effects of this problem.

Some places in the U.S. get extremely hot and humid in summer. We find that some Miniature Donkey foals do not do well in this kind of heat. They will get bouts of diarrhea, have a slight rise in temperature and may stop nursing. The average body temperature for most Miniature Donkey foals is 100-101. During these hot spells, donkey foals may develop diarrhea and have a temperature of 102. At this time you must be very certain that the foal continues to nurse. You can check this by checking the jennet's udder. If it is filled and hard to the touch, your foal has stopped nursing.

(Note: foals can take a stance beside their mothers and "appear" to be nursing. If you are not sure, get down on your knees and make sure the foal has the teat in his mouth and is sucking.) If this happens, you must immediately milk the jennet and force feed the foal. Miniature Donkey foals are so tiny that they can dehydrate in a matter of hours. Dehydration of young foals happens so fast because of the foal's small size and because the gastrointestinal system in a foal is short and doesn't reabsorb as much water as adults. Treatment for all types of serious diarrhea in foals under 30 days of age will consist of intravenous fluids, "because if they are dehydrated, the fluids go right into the bloodstream with IVs," said Dwyer. We currently treat diarrhea with a mix of 2 cc's of Pepto Bismol and 2 cc's of Kaopectate and put in a 10 cc syringe. If you use a syringe to give this mixture be sure you do not squirt it in the foal's mouth as you could choke the foal or it could go into the lungs causing pneumonia. One interesting note is that we had much more of a problem with scours before we started injecting our newborns with selenium/Vit E than we do now. We now rarely have problems with foal diarrhea. Before supplementing your foals with selenium you MUST be certain you live in a selenium deficient area of the country.

Bowel movements may vary from thin and sticky to thin and watery and of various color. Fresh bright red blood is a sign that you have a serious problem. If your foal's temperature rises above 102 and the foal looks droopy and weak and shows signs of depression, you should contact your veterinarian immediately.

Foals - especially miniatures - are small and have limited reserves of fluids and energy. They can dehydrate and become ill very quickly. If your vet suspects infection, he may take a sample of the feces to send to a lab to find out exactly which antibiotics will kill the bacteria causing the diarrhea.

However, Dwyer warns against owners reaching for a bottle of antibiotics when they discover a sick foal- "Indiscriminant use of antibiotics can complicate some diarrhea cases by lulling off 'good' bacteria in the gut. Antibiotic decisions should be left to the veterinarian." Another weapon in the arsenal to fight diarrhea is activated charcoal, which will absorb toxins that are present in the gut. The activated charcoal is a black powder that is made into a slurry with water and tubed into the foal's stomach by a veterinarian.

The foal's hind end may become scalded by the feces and you will have to cleanse the area with warm water. After it is clean, you can apply some petroleum jelly to help protect the area. This procedure should be repeated daily. It is best to not use any soap on the already irritated skin.

Foals may have diarrhea because they have been treated with antibiotics, especially if these are given orally so if your foal develops diarrhea do not automatically give it a shot of penicillin. Some drugs are more prone than others to kill off the foal's intestinal bacteria - the critters which help him to digest his food.

If the foal has diarrhea due to viral or bacterial causes, move the affected foal and its dam to a separate unit and disinfect everything in the barn from which they came. If a sick foal or foals cannot be moved to another barn, it is important to remember to care for healthy foals first, then tend to the sick ones. This helps you avoid carrying the diarrhea-causing agent from the sick foals to the healthy foals.

Reference: Bonnie Gross, Editor MDT, Ruth B. James, DVM, Roberta Dwyer, DVM

Tetanus Antitoxin

Here at Pheasant Meadow Farm, we make it our practice to attempt to be present at every birth and in fact we have missed very few as we stay on 24 hour watch. Within 15 seconds of when the navel cord breaks, we are there with the iodine and in those instances, we do not give tetanus antitoxin. However, if we are not right on the ball, or miss the birth, we give the tetanus antitoxin. Below are the feelings of two veterinarians so that you can make your own choice.

J. Warren Evans, PHD and Richard L. Torbeck, DVM: "Unless the mare has been vaccinated against tetanus within 30 days prior to foaling, the foal should be given tetanus antitoxin soon after birth. Some authorities advise that tetanus antitoxin be administered as a precautionary measure, even when the mare is on a tetanus vaccination program."

M. Phyllis Lose, VMD: "Some veterinary practitioners do not inject the tetanus antitoxin because they feel there is no need to protect the newborn foal since immunity has been scientifically proven to be available in the colostrum from the mare. However, too many variables exists that could jeopardize the foal's life if this simple protection is not provided. Because of an individual mare's peculiarity, there is always the possibility that THAT particular mare might not produce antibodies in her colostrum in spite of having received her tetanus vaccination. In addition, the known natural habitat for the tetanus spore is the feces of the horse. A newborn foal with an open navel (the best known medium for growth of spores) may struggle for hours in the manure laden straw before finally reaching its feet and successfully drinking the mare's colostrum. In my years of practice the routine injection of tetanus antitoxin to thousands of foals has yet to produce an unfavorable reaction, and of the thousands of foals injected not one has been lost from tetanus."

Tetanus Toxoid vs Tetanus Antitoxin

Update: There are two products used to prevent tetanus. One is the vaccine (or toxoid) the other is the antitoxin. The toxoid stimulates the donkey's immune system. The antitoxin provides immediate protection by supplying preformed antibodies. A change in the old recommendation of using tetanus antitoxin routinely in newborns and when wounds occur is warranted. The antitoxin can cause liver failure in a small percentage of equine several weeks to months following administration. Antitoxin should only be used in equine with wounds and no history of tetanus vaccination.

The Orphan Foal

An orphan is any foal whose mother is unwilling or unable to provide milk and/or a normal maternal relationship due to her death, illness, injury or behavioral problems. Because the newborn foal depends on its dam for immunity against infection and for the development of normal behavioral patterns, loss of the jennet during or immediately after foaling can be a serious set-back to the foal's physical and psychological development.

<u>Immediate Needs</u>

There are two categories of foals: Foals that received colostrum within 48 hours of birth and foals who did not. Colostrum gives immunity protection for 3 or 4 months and gives the orphan foal a much greater survival rate than the foal who did not receive colostrum. In some instances the jennet can be milked and bottle fed to the foal. The procedure has also been carried out successfully soon after the death of the dam.

The orphan may be strong and healthy or may be so weak that it cannot stand to nurse. A weak foal needs immediate attention to insure that it receives adequate immunity (colostrum via stomach tube or broad spectrum antibiotics) and inducement for the evacuation of its bowels. Strong orphans will usually adjust easily to being bottle fed. NOTE: Lamb nipples are the right size for donkey foals and can be found in most farm supply stores. The foal should be fed ONLY when standing or positioned over your legs in an upright position on its chest. Attempting to feed a foal who is lying down could result in milk entering the lungs, causing death.

Health Care

The orphan foal requires the same care as any newborn foal. The navel should be soaked in iodine and a tetanus antitoxin given. If colostrum was not received, an enema should be considered. Your vet may also want to administer antibiotics and vitamins. The foal's temperature is the single most important indication of its health status. A rise in temperature or a subnormal temperature are both signs of trouble.

An orphan foal is more susceptible to common foal illnesses than one raised by its mother. Diarrhea often occurs in bottle fed foals due to the high content of fat in the formula and overfeeding. Diarrhea along with colic or fever should be reported to your vet. Persistent diarrhea can significantly lower the foal's body defenses and is extremely dangerous in miniatures.

Housing is important since the foal is more sensitive to health problems. Its stall should be free from hazards as these foals are more prone to injury without their mother's supervision. In cold weather, infra-red heat lamps should be positioned in such a way that the foal can move in and out of the light freely. Foals should also be kept away from drafts.

Solid Food

The orphan should be introduced to solid feed as early as one week of age. The foal will eat very little at this time. FOAL-LAC pellets will encourage the transition from formula to grain. It is important to select a feed that is easily digestible, highly palatable, and suited to the foal's nutritional needs. Its diet should be balanced with other essential vitamins and minerals to insure proper development.

Another major concern is preparing a balanced diet for the foal is the calcium-phosphorus ratio. A correct ration (about 2:1) is essential for the development of healthy bones, joints, and tendons. Slight excesses of calcium are not detrimental, but gross excesses can cause the formation of abnormally dense, thick bone. Excess phosphorus can also cause bone problems. When excessive levels of phosphorus are present in the blood, calcium is pulled from bone to maintain the proper calcium-phosphorus ratio in the blood.

Discipline

Due to the nature of an orphan foal's upbringing, its psychological needs are just as important as its physical needs. If the foal is isolated from other donkeys, dependence on human companionship can be harmful. An ideal situation would be if you found a very friendly nurse goat who would adopt the foal from day one. The orphan should be introduced to another very friendly donkey at about one month of age. Care must be taken that the older donkey does not bully the orphan. When the foal is around two months old it can be introduced to other donkeys to adapt to rejection, intimidation and other normal behavioral patterns involved in establishing a social hierarchy. The sooner the orphan learns to become a "donkey", the easier discipline will come.

A major problem with orphans is their lack of respect for human authority. They identify human as playmates with behavior consisting of biting, kicking and rearing. As the foal becomes older, this behavior becomes dangerous. It is because of this that the foal be taught at an early age that this behavior will not be tolerated. It is equally important that the foal be allowed to romp with other foals. Biting in the very young should consist of voice discipline with a very firm "NO!" and a push. Kicking and rearing are natural play behavior but when directed towards humans, should again be corrected by voice discipline.

Feeding and Care of Orphaned Foals

- First 24 Hours
- Collection and Storage of Colostrum
- Feeding Program
- General Care
- Expected Growth Rate
- Milk Replacer for Foals

Feeding and raising orphaned foals can be an extreme challenge particularly if the foal was orphaned at birth. Losing a mare/jennet is never expected and being left with a motherless orphan can turn into an unexpected nightmare. Intensive management will optimize the foal's survival chances.

First 24 Hours

The primary concern for foals orphaned at birth must be that the foal has received sufficient amounts of colostrum. Colostrum, or a mare/jennet's first milk, contains a high concentration of immunoglobins (antibodies) to protect the foal from disease and infection. Colostrum is secreted by the mare/jennet during the first 24 to 48 hours following parturition. There is no placental transfer of antibodies during pregnancy from mare/jennet to fetus, thus the foal is born without any protection from disease. Antibodies are acquired by the nursing foal through the colostrum, (passive transfer), to protect the newborn against diseases.

Gastrointestinal tract absorption of colostrum begins to decrease after 12 hours, with minimal absorption occurring 24 hours after birth. Colostrum can be bottle fed, or administered via stomach tube by a veterinarian. A total of two to three liters of colostrum should be divided into three to four doses given at hourly intervals.

Foals that do not receive sufficient colostrum within the first 24 hours can receive blood plasma intravenously. Normal equine plasma may be purchased commercially (Foalimmune, Lake Immunogenics, Inc., Ontario, NY; Equine Plasma, Veterinary Dynamics, Inc. Chino, CA) for over $100 per liter. Intravenous infusion should be done under veterinary supervision. Plasma may be prepared locally if an acceptable donor horse/donkey and equipment are available. Without either colostrum or plasma, foals will have insufficient antibody protection and will most likely succumb to infection.

From 12 to 36 hours after birth, evaluation of the serum antibody level

(IgG) in the foal is recommended. "Failure of passive transfer" (FPT) is defined as inadequate level of antibodies or IgG of below 200 mg/dl at 24 hours of age. University of Florida studies have shown that foals with total FPT (no antibody protection) have a 75 percent chance of becoming ill. Foals with partial FPT have a 50 percent chance of becoming ill.

Several tests can be used to evaluate the antibody level in the blood of a day-old foal. New tests include radio immunodiffusion tests, latex agglutination test, and enzyme immunoassay tests (CITE). These various tests all require a small blood sample and are available from veterinarians. Regardless of the test, an IgG level of >800mg/dl is considered adequate.

Collection and Storage of Colostrum

Colostrum can be collected from mares post-foaling when sufficient amounts are present. It has been shown, 200 to 500 ml can be milked from such a mare without compromising antibody passage to her own newborn foal (125 to 175 ml for miniature donkeys). Additionally, if a mare/jennet is at risk of dying, colostrum should be harvested from her before the loss of the mare. Freezing colostrum is adequate for preservation and should have a shelf life of one year [or more] if kept frozen. Stored colostrum should be thawed at room temperature just before use. Do not thaw by microwave as essential antibodies can be destroyed.

Large broodmare farms routinely collect colostrum and freeze it to maintain a "colostrum bank" in cases of emergency. A quantitative measurement of antibody production in colostrum can be obtained by use of a colostrometer.

Feeding Program

Once sufficient immune protection has been established, some type of continued nutritional plan must begin. Normally, foals nurse up to seventeen times an hour during the first week of life. Nursing frequency decreases to three times per hour in the first few weeks of life. There are two basic options to provide sufficient nutrition to the orphaned foal -- use a nurse mare/jennet or goat, or manually feed the orphaned foal.

Obtaining a nurse mare/jennet would generally be highly desirable as it would greatly reduce labor. Unfortunately, they can be hard to find. Another potential problem includes convincing the nurse mare/jennet to accept the foal. One substitute is to use goat's milk by purchasing a milk-producing goat. Some orphan foals have been fostered onto nanny goats with minimal restraint. These goats can be placed on hay bales or platforms so the foal can nurse. As the foal grows, the goat may not provide enough milk and supplemental feed is required.

Most commonly, however, an intensive manual feeding program is developed. Initially, foals should be bottle fed either mare's milk, goat's milk, or a powdered mare's milk replacer ration. Many mare's milk replacer powders are commercially available. Also listed below are recipes for homemade milk replacers. Mare's milk replacers are preferred over milk replacers made for other species. Fresh cow's milk (whole) should be avoided. It has nearly twice as much fat content and only 2/3 the sugar content of mare's milk and generally causes loose stools in foals. Low fat cow's milk (2% fat) can be substituted for mare's milk if 20 g dextrose is added per liter. This mixture should be fed to a total volume of 10 percent of the foal's weight at one day of age and increased to 25 percent of the foals body weight from day 10 through weaning.

When bottle feeding, use of a lamb's nipple is preferred over a calf nipple, and small, frequent feedings is optimal. Very weak foals can be fed initially via nasal gastric tube (stomach tube) by a veterinarian. Foals will begin to consume solid feed within a few weeks and should have access to grain and grass or hay.

Controlling Diarrhea

A common problem with feeding orphaned foals is diarrhea. Controlling this involves manipulating the three components of a feeding program: 1) amount of milk fed per day, 2) dilution rate of the mixture, 3) number of feedings offered per day.

Amount to feed

Mares are large milkers and can produce as much as 3 percent of their body weight in milk per day. It has been shown foals can consume up to 25 percent of their body weight per day of a dilute milk replacer without risk of diarrhea. *(For miniature donkeys, see page 126 for feeding schedules.)* Foals can easily be taught to drink from a bucket at a very young age. This reduces labor needed and allows the foal to consume the milk needed.

Frequency of feedings

The number of feedings per day can affect the growth rate of an orphaned foal. The more frequently fed, the more optimal the growth rate. Foals will nurse their dams the most frequently the first week. Feeding frequency can decrease from every 1 to 2 hours the first week to every 4 to 6 hours after the second week of life. Within a few weeks of life, foals will begin solid feed consumption, allowing a fewer feedings. However, large, twice daily feedings generally produce diarrhea problems.

Dilution of milk replacer

Another important consideration is the dilution of powdered mare's milk replacer. Mare's milk contains about 10 percent dry matter (or 90% water), 2 percent protein, and 1.3 percent fat. Most milk replacers recommend a dilution rate leading to a much more concentrated milk mixture than what a foal would receive from a mare. Therefore, a much higher dilution rate (1:10), which is more similar to natural mare's milk is recommended. More diluted milk replacer solution should be fed to provide the recommended total dry matter intake.

General Care

It is essential to monitor the foal's overall health. If the mare/jennet was ill before parturition, the newborn may be malnourished. The foal should be able to stand, walk, have a suckling reflex, and nurse a bottle within two to three hours. Often times, small, weak foals may appear fine initially, but begin to deteriorate with in 24 hours. If this happens, veterinarian assistance may be critical. Foal neonatal centers are available but can be extremely expensive.

As with any newborn, a dry, clean, warm environment is essential. As the foal becomes stronger, it should be turned out into a small pasture or lot for exercise. If possible, rear the orphan with another orphan, pony, goat, or horse. Orphan foal behavior problems can be reduced if owners make every attempt to treat the foal as a horse/donkey and not as a pet.

The health care program of orphan foals must be monitored closely. All routine vaccinations and deworming must be timely for the orphan to get the greatest benefit. Foals should receive their initial vaccinations for tetanus, encephalomyelitis, influenza, and rhinopneumonitis at 60 days of age, with an additional booster four to six weeks later. Parasite control can be initiated at 60 days of age, and should be done at a minimum every eight weeks. A continuous daily dewormer is available and could benefit many orphans by minimizing parasite infestation.

Expected Growth Rate

Many believe that orphaned foals are "stunted" and never reach their genetic growth potential. However, if sufficient management is done, these foals can grow at an optimal rate. Recent research has shown orphaned foals, under intensive management and health care, were smaller and had a slower growth rate than foals suckling mares/jennets at 30 days of age. However, by 180 days of age, there was no difference in wither height, and only a slight difference in weight. Thus, with proper management, there should be no long term effects on mature size of foals orphaned at birth.

Milk Replacer for Foals

Commercial milk replacer may not always be available when needed or may be too costly for some owners. Below are several recipes for home-made milk replacers.

Formulas are to be used for a short period, when commercial mare milk replacers are unavailable:

** Table sugar may produce diarrhea and thus should be avoided

Formula 1	12 oz. 6 oz. 2 tsp.	Cow's Milk Saturated lime water dextrose **
Formula 2	2 oz. 2 oz. ½ tsp.	evaporated milk warm water white corn syrup **
Formula 3	4 oz. ½ tsp	2% cow's milk white corn syrup **

Reference: Kathy Anderson, Extension Horse Specialist

<u>Feeding The Orphan Fool</u>

Remember, the best health care plan a foal can be on, is nursing from his mother. You should never give up trying to get the mother and foal together for <u>at least 3 days</u>.

Orphan foals should be fed every two hours for the first 2 weeks, both night and day

In order of nutrition, the following ratings have been given as to #1 (best choice) on down the line.

#1 Mother's milk (you must milk the mother)
#2 Pure goats milk (many breeders have excellent experience with goats milk!)
#3 Another jennet's milk (if you nave another jennet who is nursing a foal (foal should be older than one month) who may be able to milk enough to feed the orphan, however, her own foal must have its appetite satisfied.
#4 Land 0 Lakes Mare's Milk Replacer
#5 Nutrifoal (or any other milk replacer suggested by your veterinarian)

(Foal Lac tends to give donkey foals severe diarrhea) Never use pure cow's milk.

Feed 10% or maximum of 20% of body weight of foal.

Age	**Daily Total**	**# of Feedings per Day**	**Oz per feeding**
1 day - 3 Wks	32 to 64 oz	12	3 oz to 5 oz
3 wks - 12 wks	45 to 90 oz	6	7.5 to 15 oz
l2weeks	80-l6Ooz	4	20 to 40 oz

Offer free-choice foal-lac pellets starting at 1-2 weeks of age or any other milk replacer pellet.

Imprint Training - The Newborn Foal

Foals are just as capable of learning as adult donkeys. During their first few days of life, much of the foals' future behavior and responses are shaped. The foal learns its behavior habits by observing and duplicating its mother. They also learn by using their five basic senses - new objects are spotted and carefully evaluated by sniffing and attempting to touch it. The noted Robert Miller, DVM, has worked extensively with young equine foals and has developed a technique he calls "Imprint Training". Dr. Miller believes that we can imprint certain situations into the foal's brain. He advocates working with a newborn foal as soon as possible after birth, getting it familiar with being handled and touched. This, of course, does not mean that you should invite your entire neighborhood over to handle the foal as soon as it is born. Many jennets are very nervous at this time and do not want any people around her newborn at all. If your jennet is somewhat on the nervous side, have someone halter and hold her while you are working with the foal for the first few days.

You basically want your foal to become accustomed to your smell and physical touch. Dr. Miller believes that handling and touching your foal on different parts of its body will have a lasting affect, even if it is not repeated in the near future.

He begins with the foal's head, rubbing it down and handling it all over. Each stimulus is repeated at least 30 times OR until the foal accepts it without resistance and no longer struggles but becomes relaxed. Stopping before the foal becomes relaxed does absolutely no good. The entire body of the foal is handled and rubbed.

This routine should be repeated every day for the first few days working 10 to 15 minute sessions. If you plan on showing your donkeys, this would also be a good time to get it accustomed to the sound of clippers. Handling your foal around its mouth will also make worming an easier job. Pick up its little hooves and lightly tap on them, imprinting that future trimming will not cause it pain. Try to expose the foal to everything it will encounter as an adult.

How Do Foals Learn?

Still wet and slippery, the newborn foal shakes its head and gazes at its new surroundings. Struggling to its feet, instinct guides the foal to its source of food; the jennet nuzzles him, licking and drying the furry coat. She is a show donkey, and the foal will be trained to do the same. Yet long before formal training begins, the foal has begun to learn. How does this process begin, and how can we take advantage of what we know to produce a well mannered adult?

One big difference between the young donkey and the young human or dog is the foal's relative independence at birth. While humans are born helpless and totally dependent upon their parents, the foal is born "precocious," able to fend for itself to a greater extent. Because they're born with all systems fully developed, foals are just as capable of learning as an adult donkey.

Human babies spend several years going through the various stages of learning (or "critical handling periods," as the scientists say), but the foal probably has a crash course beginning in the first few days of its life. During this time period, much of the foal's future behavior and responses are shaped, and the foal is most amenable to new experiences. This was necessary for survival of donkeys in the wild, as they had to be able to follow their mother and to escape from predators at a very early age.

The first few hours of a foal's life are spent taking care of the basic need for nourishment. The normal foal, acting purely from instinct, attempts to stand and nurse shortly after birth. This process involves some trial and error, as the foal stands, topples over, and again struggles to its feet. The search for the teat may take awhile, but eventually is successful. Although we may be tempted to assist, it's usually best to stand back and watch. Dr. Sharon Crowell-Davis, a behavior specialist at the University of Georgia, comments in the Equine Practice Journal, "This searching is more than just a means to an end. It is a process by which the foal learns about its mother – the topography and odors which serve as cues for where to seek milk, and who to stay near. Human intervention to move a normal, healthy foal directly onto the teat as soon as it stands up interrupts this learning process."

The foal learns his behavior habits, from grazing to sexual behavior, by observing and copying his mother and other donkeys. Deprived of this opportunity to interact with others of his own kind, he may not know what to do later on. (Many a young stallion, confused about his duties, has been cured by watching an older stallion at work.) Foals also learn by using their other senses: touch, taste, and hearing. New objects are evaluated by careful sniffing and an occasional attempt at tasting them.

Equine operate in a world of dominance and submission. The foal quickly learns his place in the herd by the actions of his companions. Once you've established yourself as the dominant member of your partnership, all further interactions are made much easier. If this relationship isn't clear, the equine will challenge everything you do, putting itself and you in a dangerous position.

Starting training with the young foal has several advantages. Younger foals are quicker learners than their older counterparts. The foal is small and easily handled; this reduces the risk of injury for both the handler and the donkey.

Most of our mastery over the donkey or horse is psychological. We can teach the foal to be submissive before it is able to use its size to take advantage of the situation. How do you do this? It's easy with the young foal: Simply hold it until it stops struggling; a daily dose of this will show him that you're the one in control of the situation. Bad habits like nipping and rearing can (and should) be stopped before they become dangerous. Of course, there are plenty of adult equine out there who were not trained at an early age and are still fine to work with now. The point is that the training period will be that much easier and safer for all, avoiding future fights and extended workouts, if it's begun early.

Equine are naturally timid animals and have always been the prey in a world of predators. Most of the animals' reactions which annoy us are the result of fear and their attempts to escape what they view as a threatening situation. Equine are also very intelligent animals; we can teach them to overcome that fear and behave in a more desirable way. Although the equine has a very limited ability to reason, it has high learning and memory abilities. One of the easiest ways to teach a donkey is the process of habituation, or flooding. This simply means getting a donkey used to something new by exposing him to it frequently, until he accepts the situation. For this process to work, the donkey must not be able to escape or avoid the situation.

DVM Robert Miller, a California veterinarian, has worked extensively with young foals and has developed a technique he calls imprint training. The imprinting period of a foal is that time early in life when events most strongly affect the foal's behavior and when it's most receptive to information. This does not mean that you, the neighbors, and all the kids should go into the stall at the moment of birth to habituate the foal to people! Many a foal which the vet had to check because it "just won't nurse" was suffering from a simple case of too many people causing too much confusion.

Common sense should dictate how and when you work with your new foal. While some jennets and mares will accept the presence of people shortly after foaling, others may become extremely nervous, and may even be dangerous. Too much interference by too many people during the time shortly after the foal's birth may be detrimental to the initiation of nursing and other interactions between the jennet and foal.

In her article, Dr. Crowell-Davis points out: "Foals begin life with a predisposition to follow any large, moving object. Thus, correct imprinting on their own mother requires some degree of isolation of the foal and its mother from other large moving objects, i.e., other donkeys and people. Human handling, except for medical necessities, should be avoided during the first day of life, in order to avoid disruption of imprinting on the mother."

Dr. Bonnie Beaver, a behaviorist at Texas A&M University, points out that the critical imprinting stage probably can go on for at least the first several days of life. "The concept of working with the foal, getting it to know your smell, getting it used to actually being physically dominated...is best done during the imprinting stage, certainly within a few days of birth." Dr. Beaver doesn't think that mare-foal imprinting will be adversely affected by the presence of people. "We know that even in situations where the mare has died at birth, the foal will still imprint on its own species, is capable of identifying and separating out individuals at that time."

While the scientists' viewpoint may seem impersonal to some, it's just a rephrasing of what many trainers have known and practiced for years: Frequent, early handling of the foal made its future training that much easier.

Safety and the health of the foal should be of the utmost importance. Be sure there is someone present to hold the jennet while you are working with the foal; it helps to have a handler for the foal as well, so that you can go through your routine more easily. The jennet and foal will be more relaxed if they're held nose to nose during their handling.

Remember all the senses, including smell, sound, and touch and think of all the problems you've ever had working with donkeys and horses: clipping their ears, taking a temperature, cleaning the prepuce, opening their mouths. Habituating the foal to these procedures may make future procedures much easier!

Take advantage of the foals' small size to accustom it to handling while it still can't fight back or escape. This isn't a torture session, though. It should be a pleasant experience for the foal; after initial resistance, the rubdown starts to feel good! Like all animals, foals like to be touched.

Whether or not you're present at the moment of birth, this type of routine can be done each day for the first few days of the foal's life. Short attention spans can be accommodated by working in brief, 15 minute sessions. The important point is to start handling early, to take advantage of both the "critical learning period" and the foal's small size.

Although the younger foal is most highly receptive to learning, the procedure can still be followed on the older foal. It's vital that the foal not be able to escape or avoid each stimulus (because then you're just teaching him to escape!) and that the exposure continue until the foal accepts the procedure quietly.

After this initial introduction to the variety of life, you can get your foal off to a quick start on what otherwise might be some difficult situations. This includes anything which might be seen as frightening, but is non-painful. trailering, haltering, standing tied, and tolerating clippers are all within the realm of the 1- to 2-week old foal. Keep your lessons short to accommodate the foals' brief concentration span, and don't overwhelm him with too many different things at once.

Having a jennet who tolerates all these procedures makes life easier; you can lead the jennet into a trailer and the foal usually follows without hesitation. Taking the pair for short walks while you have time and patience will save hours of frustration some day in the future when you need to get somewhere in a hurry.

You can accustom your foal to clippers without actually clipping him; simply turn them on, and leave them outside the stall for a few minutes each day. While someone holds the foal, hold the clippers up against his body, along his legs, and near his ears. Continue this until he relaxes and begins to ignore you.

The possibilities are endless; imagine how much easier this foal will be to train as a yearling and 2-year old! The lesson is simple: Expose the foal to everything he'll experience as an adult, do it in short, daily lessons, and do it early. Your veterinarian will love you when worming goes off without a fight and the teeth get floated with the donkey's head in a normal position. You'll be happier, getting things done without tranquilizers or a twitch, and everyone will have far less risk of injury.

Reference: Dr. Carin Smith has been a practicing veterinarian since 1984.

The Dead Foal

Not a popular subject, but one that we all need to know about. The following comments are from M. Phyllis Lose, V.M.D.

"Every year, unfortunately, some foals are born dead. Veterinary examination of the carcass via a postmortem can and usually does provide answers as to the probable cause of death. This information can be more complete and somewhat more sophisticated when the service of a veterinary pathologist is engaged.

A great deal of practical (basic) information concerning the plight of the emerging foal can be gleaned by reading the color, texture and consistency of the oral and ocular (eye) membranes. The shorter the time span between delivery and examination, the more accurate the evaluation. Ideally, the postmortem should take place immediately after delivery.

The color of the membranes alone can denote approximately when, and where in the reproductive tract, death occurred. When the membranes are a dark, muddy color, it is suggestive of intrauterine death (inside the uterus) from one of many causes. Regardless of the cause, death assuredly ensued in the uterus well in advance of delivery, perhaps from 12 to 24 hours prior to delivery. The dead foal has remained in the uterus long enough for the lack of circulation to create tissue changes causing a foreign-body reaction in the dam, and abortion or delivery of a deal foal.

Other color variations, from the extremes of very white to darker shades, tell us that most likely the foal perished very close to the time of delivery or actually during delivery. Darkened bluish or reddish membranes indicate a recent death by failure of the oxygen and nutritional support systems. These individuals perish in the uterus and are subsequently delivered post-haste, or have died in the reproductive canal, or advanced as far as the vagina and then expired.

In foals with startling snow-white membranes, the limbs of these foals are invariably icy cold. Other dead foals, following delivery, are normally warm from the mare's internal body temperature. This departure from the expected would appear to indicate a shock-like syndrome. In each of these cases, I was able to establish that the foal was unusually active in utero, kicking strongly or even violently just prior to delivery as if the intrauterine death was of a frantic, convulsive nature. This activity leads me to consider the possibility of sudden mechanical physiologic failure."

(Ed Note: If you discover a jennet in labor and the nose and legs are there, however, feel cold, don't assume that the baby is dead. The baby could have kicked just a minute for two before you discovered the jennet and the sac broke. In just a minute, the wet legs will feel cold to the touch. Just about all foals are born with their tongues hanging out of their mouths while they are in the birth canal. They look dead, but that's the way the all look! Whether the foal is dead or not, it is still extremely urgent that you get the foal out for the sake of the jennet. I have noticed a dramatic difference between horse mares and donkey jennets. I find that horse mares are likely to abort a non-viable or diseased fetus much earlier in pregnancy. Donkey jennets, unfortunately, tend to carry these same foals, much longer and closer to full term. It is difficult to tell if an aborted donkey fetus at 9, 10, or 11 months if full term or not if the owner is not aware of an actual breeding date as all the parts will be there and the fetus will have plenty of hair.)

Chapter 7

Foal Illness and Disease

Weak Flexor Tendons in the Miniature Donkey Newborn

A normal feature of newborn foals is some degree of lax ligaments or flaccid flexor tendons in all four legs. This "down at the pasterns" appearance places the fetlocks closer to - sometimes even touching - the ground, in severe cases as the one shown at the right. The condition is present at birth and is most common in the rear legs but may occur in all four legs. In severe cases, the fetlock area *only* should be bandaged to prevent abrasion. These loose ligaments tighten up with age and activity in a relatively short time. Usually within a few days or weeks, the pasterns will achieve a steeper angle, and the fetlocks will be higher off the ground.

The mother and foal should always be separated from the rest of the herd. Mothers are very protective of their newborns, and a foal that cannot move very quickly could easily be injured in a scuffle. Treatment will consist of both rest and <u>limited</u> exercise however, the pair should not be kept in a stall. The foal needs to move around in a small paddock area to help strengthen the ligaments, <u>yet</u> should not be continuously running which may cause further weakness due to strain.

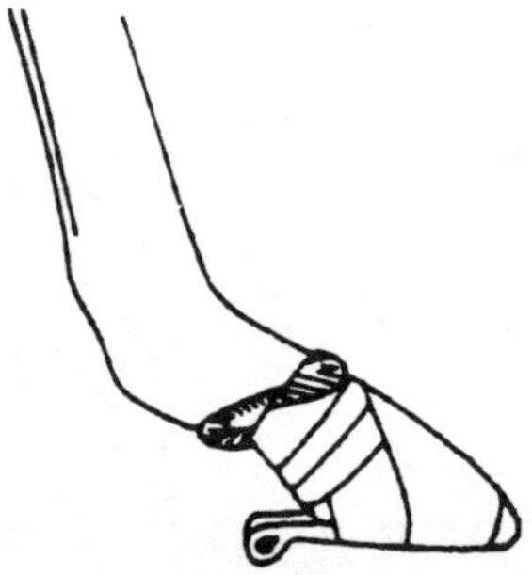

If little or no improvement is seen in seven days, the foot may be fitted with a trailer shoe applied with surgical adhesive tape. The rear extension helps to support the foal's foot and forces the toe downward.

Casting the legs is *never* an option nor is hard bandaging. Casting causes muscles and tendons to lose strength thus the condition could be twice as bad as it started out and even require that the animal be put down.

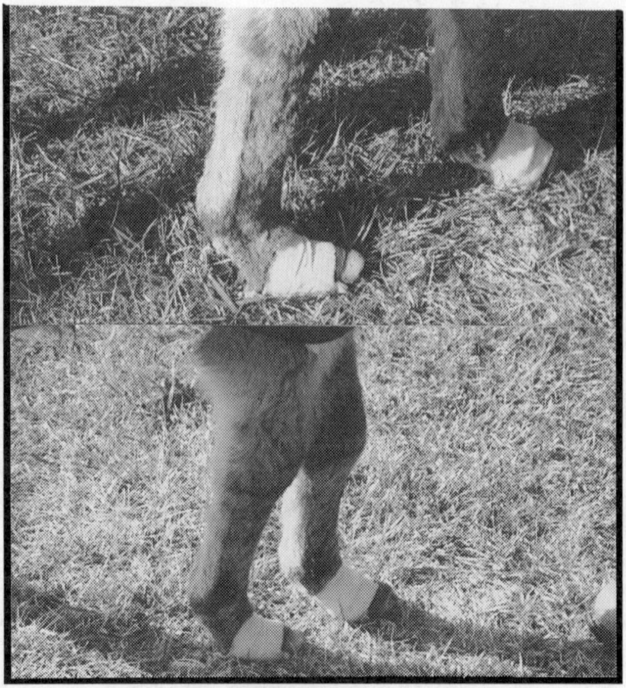

Day One

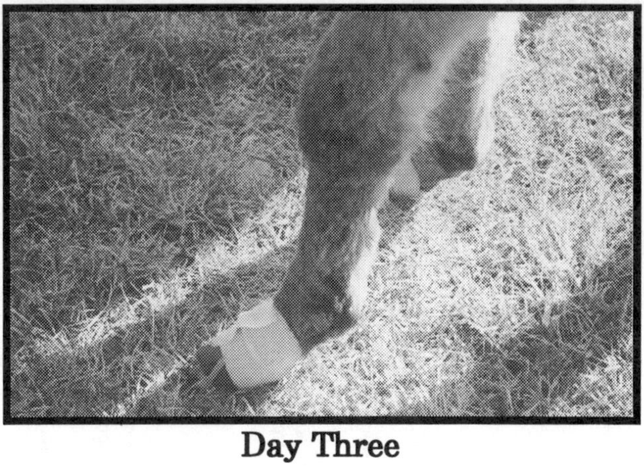

Day Three

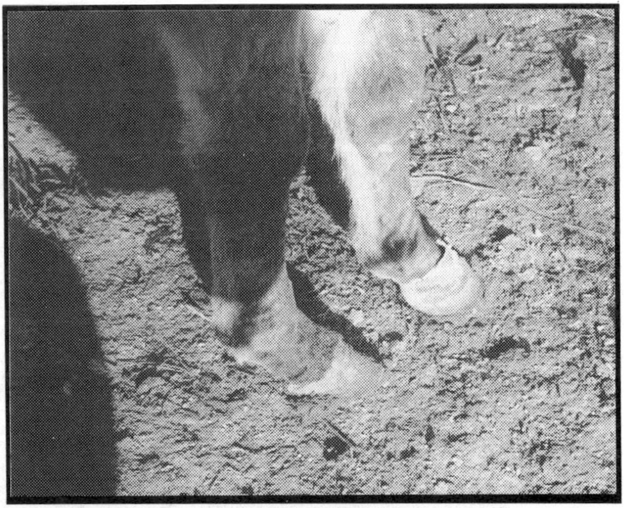

Day Six

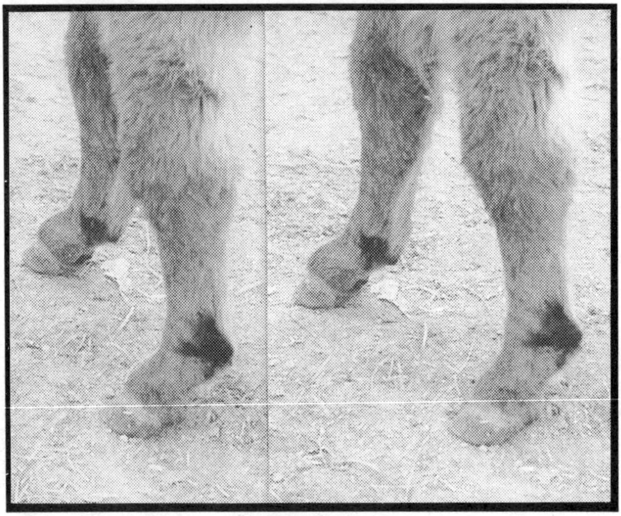

Day Nine

Hernias

A hernia is the protrusion of an organ or tissue through the wall of a cavity that normally contains the organ or tissue. In foals, two types of hernias occur with some degree of frequency: umbilical and scrotal hernias.

Umbilical hernias result when a section of intestine protrudes through the umbilical opening in the abdominal wall. Normally, this opening constricts shortly after birth, but occasionally closure is delayed. If a piece of intestine becomes displaced through this opening, a lump is usually observed in the navel area. Although the bowel often becomes repositioned and the opening usually closes within one year; surgical closure is required in some cases. It is important to note that the opening may close around a piece of intestine, cutting off the blood supply to the displaced tissue. When bowel strangulation occurs, the foal initially becomes listless and only later shows signs of colic. Bowel strangulation requires surgical correction.

Scrotal hernias occur in males when a piece of intestine is displaced through the inguinal canal (the pathway for the descending testes) and into the scrotum. (If the intestine is lodged in the inguinal canal, it is referred to as an inguinal hernia.) The affected colt may show signs of intestinal pain or altered gait and usually has scrotal swelling. Like the umbilical hernia, this condition is usually corrected naturally, but the possibility of bowel strangulation is always a concern. Scrotal hernias may be congenital or acquired; although when such a hernia is seen in very young foals, the condition is thought to be congenital. Because the condition is also thought to be heritable, these animals are usually castrated.

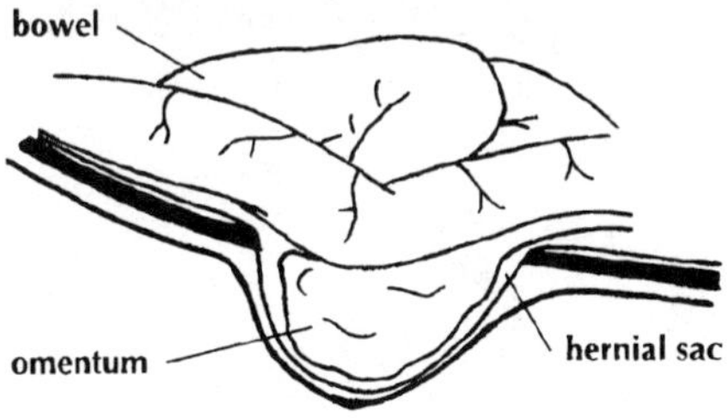

Rotavirus In Foals

If not dealt with properly, this intestinal pathogen can cause serious problems for many years.

Diarrhea in foals is always a serious situation, except for the temporary looseness of stool during the jennet's first heat cycle. Foals can dehydrate rapidly when they suffer from infectious diarrhea, and the dehydration can be fatal. The diarrhea can be caused by a number of things, including improper nutrition, dirt-eating, parasites, bacteria, viruses or stressful conditions such as bad weather. Most of the more serious types of foal diarrhea are caused by infectious organisms, and a rotavirus is one of the most common villains.

The rotavirus is an intestinal pathogen and is found in many environments where there are many donkeys (especially foals); it is a common problem on breeding farms. The rotavirus is fairly tough and aggressive, and seems to attack a foal's intestinal lining even without prior damage or irritation to

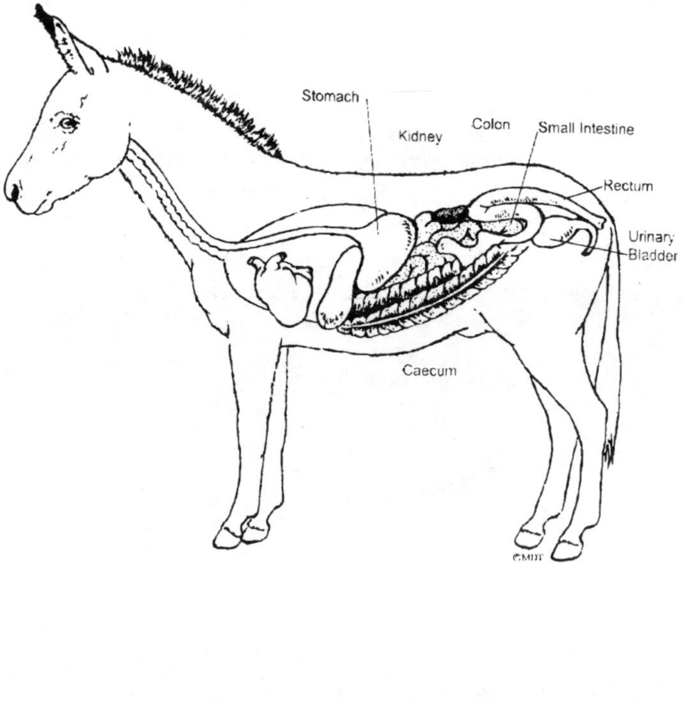

the gut caused by bacteria or parasites. Some viruses are opportunistic invaders that attack only after an animal's resistance has been lowered by stress or the tissues have been weakened from prior infection by bacteria or some other invader. But the rotavirus marches right in and starts the attack on its own.

This virus seems to persist on a farm almost indefinitely once it is established there (usually brought in with a new animal or introduced by someone - on their feet or clothing - who was recently on a farm already contaminated with this virus). The virus lurks in the barnyard and stalls to cause new infections and may persist for years, infecting each new foal crop.

Rotavirus diarrhea usually hits foals anytime from birth up to a month of age and comes on swiftly. This is the age when the foal's immature immune system has not yet had a chance to develop defenses against many of the pathogens in the surrounding environment. After one month, most foals have stronger defenses and are not as easily felled by this type of infection.

When the foal becomes sick with rotavirus infection, he may have a fever and appear depressed for a few hours, then breaks with diarrhea. These foals are usually quite dull and sick, in contrast to the foal experiencing "foal heat" diarrhea that stays lively and bright and usually keeps his appetite and vigor. The foal with rotavirus diarrhea passes runny bowel movements that may be of a cow-pie consistency or looser (watery), and the feces will be yellowish-green to gray. If the feces are quite loose and watery, the foal may dehydrate very rapidly due to loss of important body fluids.

Much of the fluid and nutrients that the foal eats and drinks are absorbed by the small intestine; the lining is a special "doorway" where the fluid and nutrients can go into the bloodstream to be moved around the body to wherever needed. The surface of the small intestinal lining is made up of tiny finger-like projections called villi. This "shag-carpet" effect gives the intestine a tremendous increase in total surface area for absorption.

Each finger-like projection of the lining is thickly covered with even smaller, microscopic villi that absorb the fluid and nutrients corning through the intestine from the stomach, and many of these tiny villi host a number of special enzymes that break down complex sugars into simpler sugars that can be more easily digested and absorbed. One of the most important enzymes produced by the microvilli is lactase, which breaks down the milk sugar lactose. The foal must have this enzyme to digest and absorb his mother's milk.

When a rotavirus infects the foal's digestive tract, it sets up shop in the small intestine and begins damaging and destroying the microvilli. This interferes with the digestive enzymes, and the foal can no longer digest milk. So the first result of the rotavirus infection is many undigested sugars and fats passing through the intestines instead of being broken down and absorbed. As these undigested particles pass through the large intestine, they irritate its lining, causing the foal's body to secrete more fluid and electrolytes into the large intestine to try to wash out the irritation and move it out of the tract.

But this doesn't work very well and actually creates a double problem for the foal. The increased fluid secretion into the large intestine makes his feces runny and watery, and the decreased absorption ability of the gut lining makes it impossible for him to replace this lost fluid. His body tissues begin to dehydrate. He can become seriously ill in just a few hours - the dehydration can kill him. His eyes start to look sunken, his legs become cold due to decreased blood circulation, etc. The extra fluid in and around his cells and in his bloodstream pulled out of his body and poured out through the large intestine due to the irritation in his gut. Even if he is still nursing or if you give him extra oral fluids, his damaged intestinal lining can't absorb enough - it just goes through. If his gut lining is already seriously damaged, it doesn't do any good to give him extra fluids by mouth or stomach tube for he can't absorb them.

If the foal is sick but not yet dehydrated (and his feces are not yet watery), his gut lining may not be too damaged - and you can give him oral fluids (water and electrolytes by nursing bottle or stomach tube) to prevent dehydration and replace what he is losing. Electrolytes and glucose in the water (simplest form of these important minerals and nutrients) can be absorbed without having to be digested.

But if he is feverish and passing watery feces with extensive gut-lining damage already, he won't be able to absorb enough fluid and nutrients through the digestive tract and should be started on intravenous fluids immediately. He probably won't feel like nursing and will need intensive care and supportive treatment like IVs to keep him going and help him recover.

Actually , his milk intake should be reduced for about 36 to 48 hours if he has severe diarrhea to keep from irritating the damaged digestive tract further and to give it a chance to start healing. Foals with severe diarrhea and intestinal damage will recover faster if they are taken completely off milk for a short time so the gut is no longer irritated and can start to heal.

In a severe case of diarrhea, take the foal off milk for at least a day (and milk the jennet at regular intervals to keep up her flow) and give him electrolyte fluids orally and/or intravenously. Antibiotics are no help in eradicating the rotavirus, but they can be given to prevent or halt secondary bacterial infection that may be causing complications.

Rotavirus diarrhea is very contagious and can go through an entire foal crop unless precautions are taken to keep it from spreading through the herd. Stalls should be thoroughly cleaned out and disinfected between foalings and occupants if donkeys must be moved. Actually, the less rotation of animals through the stalls and paddocks, the less chance of spreading problems. Farms where jennets foal out in their own stalls or paddocks usually have much less incidence of foal diarrhea than do farms where the jennets are all put through foaling stalls. Using the same stalls for a number of different jennets or jennets and foals seems to greatly increase the risk of spreading the infectious diarrhea through the group.

The rotavirus is present in the feces of a foal two days before he actually breaks with diarrhea and for up to five days after he gets over the diarrhea. Therefore a foal can infect other foals even when he himself has no symptoms. If he is coming down with the intestinal infection, he may infect other foals or contaminate a stall or paddock even before you know he is sick. During this time period just before and just after the actual diarrhea, the foal is shedding millions of pathogenic organisms into the environment. The convalescing foal that is no longer scouring should not be put with other jennets and foals; the pair should be kept separate in isolation for a safe period of time after the foal seems to be recovering.

On breeding farms where outbreaks of rotavirus diarrhea have occurred, strict isolation of sick babies and their mothers and thorough disinfecting of contaminated areas seem to help slow down the spread of diarrhea through the rest of the foals. Iodine is a good disinfectant against rotavirus, as are the phenols (a group of strong-smelling chemicals derived from coal tar and quite poisonous). Some of the more common and milder disinfectants do not inactivate the rotavirus, especially in the presence of organic matter such as straw, hay, manure, etc.

On breeding farms where rotavirus is a problem, the best preventative measure seems to be strict hygiene. The people who attend foalings and care for the foals should diligently resort to frequent hand washings, use protective clothing (one set of coveralls or overclothing when handling the sick ones that can be taken off so that no contamination on clothing is carried from sick donkeys to healthy ones, etc.) and feet rinsing in disinfectant foot baths between stalls. This way the virus won't be tracked or carried from stall to stall. This can really help in cutting down the spread of diarrhea among the foals.

Rotavirus is a deadly killer of foals, but good management on breeding farms and careful attention to cleanliness along with alert detection of early sickness, isolation and proper treatment of scouring foals - can do much toward preventing losses from this culprit.

Reference: Written by Heather Smith Thomas

Equine Tapeworms

Unwelcome and unannounced they come, developing silently within the intestines of the horse. Within the cecum, the parasites usually surround

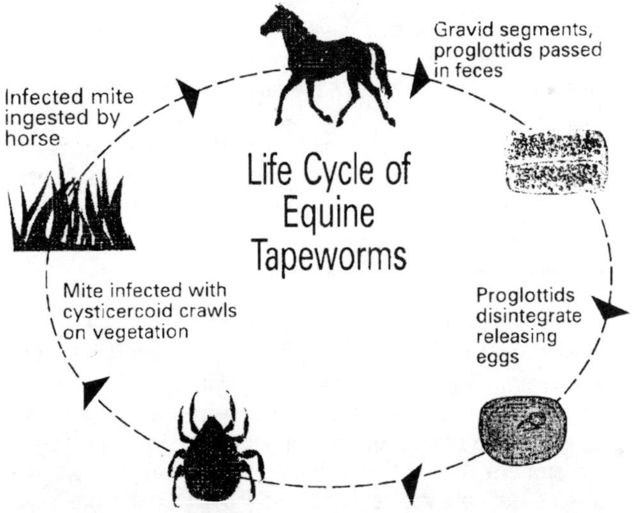

the ileocecal valve. Having no mouth parts or digestive tract, they absorb nutrients through their cuticle. The equine tapeworm can grow to about 3 inches long by 1/2 inch wide. Its head, called a scolex, has four suckers that attach to the mucosa or lining of the intestine; below each sucker is a tiny flap called a lappet. Recent surveys in horses at necropsy in Central Kentucky revealed a prevalence rate of nearly 60%.

Tapeworms are a member of the group of parasites called flatworms, which also includes flukes. The tapeworm are referred to as cestodes.

There are three species in the United States, Anoplocephala perfoliata, Anoplocephala magna, and Paranoplocephala mamillana.

Tapeworm segments (proglottids) contain both male and female organs. Proglottids progress through development from immature, mature, adult, and gravid. This last segment contains fertile eggs, sloughs off and passes in the manure as shown in Figure 1. An intermediate host, an oribatid or free-living mite found on pastures, eats the tapeworm eggs which undergo a period of development of two to four months inside the mite before reaching the infective or cysticercoid stage. For a donkey to become infected with a tapeworm, it must, as it grazes, ingest mites containing the immature or cysticercoid stage of the parasite. The chances of a donkey becoming infected are high because there are millions of oribatid mites in pasture.

Aside from the usual clinical signs of parasitism (e.g., unthriftiness, rough haircoat, lethargy, loss of appetite, diarrhea), it is very difficult to diagnose tapeworm infection. This is because the parasites do not lay eggs that can be readily detected by examining a fecal sample. Eggs present in the feces are the result of a ruptured proglottid.

Tapeworms are usually viewed as benign when compared with some of the other parasites. However, heavy infections can result in cecal hemorrhaging, blockage, ulcers, perforation, and have been suspected of causing hypermotility within the intestine.

Farm managers, owners, and veterinarians who worm exclusively with the avermectin-types (ivermectin and moxidectin) are not addressing the tapeworm problem. These dewormers have no activity against tapeworms. Pyrantel has been proven to be active against equine tapeworms, but unfortunately, there is no compound currently on the market labeled as such. Until a commercial product can be developed for the removal of cestodes, concerned individuals should discuss appropriate methods of treatment with their veterinarians.

The Parasitology Section at the Gluck Equine Research Center is continuing to monitor the prevalence of tapeworms in Kentucky horses and has an ongoing program of drug-testing to find a cestocide that is efficacious and economical.

Reference: Maxwell H. Gluck Equine Research Center Lexington, Kentucky

Navel Ill

This is a disease problem seen in young foals, which result from infection entering through the umbilical cord (navel). In some instances, the bacteria causing the problem may enter through the digestive tract. It occurs in foals from a few days to three or four months old.

An abscess at the stump of the umbilicus may be the first sign. The area becomes hot and swollen and may be discolored to bluish or purple. Sometimes, there may be no signs at the navel and the foal will be noticed to be severely lame. This may be bad enough that he is walking on three legs, and the owner immediately assumes that he has been kicked. Do NOT assume that he has been injured by the mare! Call your veterinarian immediately!

The lameness is generally accompanied by a fever (up to 101.5 degrees F or more (38.5 degrees C). The foal may be depressed. The pulse may be weak and rapid and the mucous membranes injected (reddened). Several joints may be swollen, showing that the bacterial infection has localized there. The fetlock, hip, stifle, and elbow joints are most commonly affected. The joints may feel hot to the touch and the foal may show severe pain if they are forcibly moved. The white blood count (WBC) is elevated. X-rays may be necessary to determine the extent of the damage to the joint. If left untreated, severe damage to the joint surface may occur and the animal may be permanently crippled.

Treatment includes antibiotics recommended by your veterinarian. These are usually administered for a MINIMUM of five to seven days. If treatment is started before damage to the joint cartilage has occurred, the foal may be much improved within 24 hours and will be nursing. The temperature will return to normal. Do NOT stop treatment at this time or the infection will come back. This time you will have pure pus in the joints. When the antibiotics are used for only three days, they will clear the bacteria from the blood stream (this is why the foal feels so much better). This length of time is inadequate to remove them from the joints.

Consult a veterinarian for a foal with joint or navel ill. Owner treatment, especially if inadequate in quantity or duration, may complicate the problem and lead to a joint ill that cannot be cured. Some foals may require surgery to help remove damaged tissue from the joint surface and bone. In some severe cases, the joint cartilage is damaged beyond repair and the foal will never be normal. In these cases, euthanasia is recommended for humane reasons.

In some cases, a procedure called joint lavage is used. This involves anesthetizing the foal and putting two large needles into opposite sides of an affected joint. Tubes are attached to the needles and a pump is used to flush antibiotic or other cleansing solutions through the joint cavity. Incidentally, the same procedure is sometimes used in older animals to remove cartilage debris and other material which is causing destruction within a joint. If an abscess at the navel is the only problem, it may be necessary to open and drain it. Leave this to your veterinarian and follow his instructions for aftercare religiously.

Foal Septicemia

This is an infection which becomes spread throughout the foal's bloodstream. It may be due to bacteria, viruses, or a fungus. It may originate within the uterus before birth, or may enter the foal through the digestive tract, lungs, or umbilical cord. It is most common in foals with poor immune systems, premature foals, or those less than two weeks old. A mare who drips milk prior to foaling may lose all her colostrum by the time the foal is born resulting in a lack of antibodies. It is also seen in foals who do not receive any colostrum. Management problems, such as damp, drafty quarters, overcrowding, and filth, may make the foal more susceptible. However, it can occasionally occur under the best of conditions. A septicemia may result in an animal's death or leave it with a chronic infection, stunted, or a poor-doer.

The foal may be lethargic or depressed, even comatose. He may not be nursing, leaving the mare's udder bulging and painful. His mucous membranes may be bright red to purple. The foal may be in shock. He may be jaundiced (yellow). There may be small hemorrhages inside the mouth and ears. Nervous system signs may be seen, especially coma or convulsions. The foal may show dehydration. When the skin in pinched and released, it will stand up where it has been pinched together. Check the foal's umbilical cord for swelling or drainage of urine. He mayor may not have diarrhea. Joint ill - with its hot, painful, swollen joints - may accompany the septicemia.

Foal septicemia is VERY serious and often fatal. Call your veterinarian immediately if you suspect this problem. Prompt, intensive treatment is the only thing that will save the foal. Even with the best of care, the problem is so intense that many foals are lost. Your veterinarian will treat for shock and for the organisms causing the disease.

Prevention involves management to reduce stress to the foal. Foaling quarters should be clean, warm, and dry. Make sure that the foal gets colostrum. If you have reason to suspect that the mare has none, try to get some from another mare or use some that you have frozen from a normal mare. Foals from mares who have previously had problems may need preventive antibiotics for a few days. The mare should be kept up on her immunizations to keep up the degree of immunity that she passes on to her foal. The umbilical cord should be disinfected with iodine more than once. Do it right after the foal is born, and at least once or twice more, 12 to 24 hours later. On some premises, the umbilical stump is iodined daily for five to seven days.

A Deadly Cough
The Seriousness of Foal Pneumonia

Rhodococcus equi pneumonia in the foal can be deadly, but good management could save the day.

When foals get sick, owners can sometimes face many sleepless nights, as well as weeks or months of intensive management, to get these babies through the rough spots. One of the most common problems in the ill foal is pneumonia, caused by a bacteria called Rhodococcus equi, which attacks foals between one and six months of age. Most foals will tend to show clinical signs, including coughing, abnormal breathing patterns and, less commonly, diarrhea, before the age of four months. Most farms are susceptible to the disease, but some farms are considered enzootic or particularly prone to continually have the problem. On these enzootic farms, the disease can lead to significant financial loss because of the cost of therapy and the occasional death of foals.

While adult can carry R. equi in small numbers in their intestine and not suffer any ill effects, in the foal, the organism can actually multiply in the intestine for up to three months of age so that the presence of foals inevitably contributes to the development of the infection on the farm. Foals with R. equi pneumonia swallow the mucous that accompanies the illness, the bacteria ends up back in their intestines. Therefore, their manure is likely a major source of contamination. Under suitable conditions of high summer temperatures, R. equi can multiply in the environment by 10,000-fold in only two weeks. A single gram of soil contaminated with foal manure may therefore, under favorable conditions, contain millions of virulent R. equi. The inhalation of dust particles laden with virulent R. equi. is the major route of pneumonic infection in foals.

The successful control of R. equi infections on the enzootic farm depends on several factors: decreasing the size of the infective challenge, earlier recognition of the disease and passive immunization.

Decreasing the size of infective challenge

There is a progressive buildup of infection on farms whose business it is to handle broodmares and foals. Enzootic farms are therefore likely to be those used for breeding animals for many years, those with heavy concentrations of mares and foals, and those located where summer temperatures are high, where soil type is sandy and where dust is extensive. Enzootically affected farms are usually easily recognized as those where the loafing paddocks have been turned into grassless dusty sand pits. Keeping large numbers of foals on bare, dusty, manure-containing paddocks will result in heavy challenge, with clinical disease maintaining virulent bacteria.

It is important to house foals in well ventilated, dust-free areas and to avoid dirt paddocks and crowding. Pneumonic foals must be isolated because they are the major source of contamination of the environment with virulent organisms and their manure must be composted. Pastures must be rotated to decrease dust formation and consequent inhalation of R. equi. Any sandy or dirt areas should ideally be planted with grass and made off limits to foals, or alternatively, irrigation may be useful in decreasing dust formation and encouraging grass. Manure should be regularly removed from paddocks and composted. Because mares and foals tend to congregate around water sources and under shade in hot summers, a reduction in the size of mare and foal bands may reduce destruction of grass and exposure to barren soil.

The environmental growth of R. equi increases progressively with temperatures to 86 degrees after which it plateaus. Immunization of mares and foals against common respiratory viral agents (influenza, equine herpesvirus types 1 and 4), an effective parasite control program, and adequate colostrum intake with detection and treatment of cases of failure of passive transfer may help by preventing potential predisposing illnesses.

Earlier recognition of the disease R. equi pneumonia is often not recognized until it is well-advanced and, therefore, difficult to treat. Even severely affected foals may appear to a casual observer to suck and behave normally. Early recognition of the disease with isolation and appropriate treatment of infected foals will reduce losses, limit the spread of virulent organisms in the environment and decrease the cost of therapy.

Careful weekly physical examination and auscultation of the lungs by a veterinarian is successful in promoting early diagnosis of pneumonia, therefore reducing mortality. Another approach said to be helpful in early diagnosis is testing foals from birth to five months of age at two-week intervals with the agar-gel immunodiffision (AGID) assay. The AGID test mainly detects precipitating antibody against enzypes produced by R. equi. However, a few foals may develop R. equi pneumonia without developing enough antibody to be detected by AGID and many foals will produce antibody from exposure to R. equi in their environment without subsequently developing the disease. For this reason, a combination of careful daily observations and temperature recording, as well as AGID testing or measurement of fibrinogen concentrations at two week intervals, although labor intensive, may prove to be the best approach to early identification of pneumonic foals on enzootic farms.

On such farms, routine ultrasonographic examination of the lungs by a veterinarian is another sensitive method that may allow early detection of lung lesions before development of clinical signs. Ultrasound is also helpful to evaluate response to therapy. A combination of the diagnostic tests presented here will allow early identification of foals with pneumonia. However, the only definitive way to confirm R. equi, as opposed to other bacterial pathogens, really is the cause of the infection, is bacteriologic culture of tracheal or bronchial fluid. The distinction between pneumonia caused by R. equi and that caused by other bacterial pathogens in important because the treatment approaches are different.

Passive immunization

Passive immunization with the intravenous administration of hyperimmune (HI) plasma has become a popular and generally effective way to reduce the incidence of and deaths resulting from R. equi on enzootic farms. Although time consuming to administer and expensive to produce or buy, this is the single most cost-effective measure to prevent the disease on farms with a high incidence of R. equi pneumonia.

Active immunization

It would be considerably more convenient to control R. equi pneumonia on enzootically infected farms by the active immunization of mares and their foals with a protective antigen rather than by the intravenous administration of a large volume of plasma. Such experimental attempts have been generally unrewarding and vaccines against R. equi infections are not currently available.

Clearly, R. equi can be a devastating and demoralizing problem on some farms. Control is possible, but expensive. It is also crucial that pneumonic foals are not sent to spread infection from enzootic farms to those farms with little contamination. Improved and less expensive control approaches in the long term will depend on a better understanding of why this disease attacks the young foal.

Reference: AAEP Reprinted with permission. Author: Steve Giguére, DVM, Diplomate ACVIM, and John F. Prescott, VetMB, PhD He presented his findings during the 1997 AAEP Convention in Phoenix, Arizona.

Normal and Abnormal Foal Legs

- When are the young foals legs considered too crooked and when are they within acceptable limits?
- What hoof angles are considered abnormal and need correction and when are they best left alone?
- When is the time to call a veterinarian or a farrier experienced in hoof and leg correction?
- When is the best time for a foal's first trim - in three or four weeks or three or four months?

The concerned foal owner will need a highly skilled farrier and a knowledgeable veterinarian to aid them in dealing with hoof and leg problems. The three of you must first determine if there is a problem.

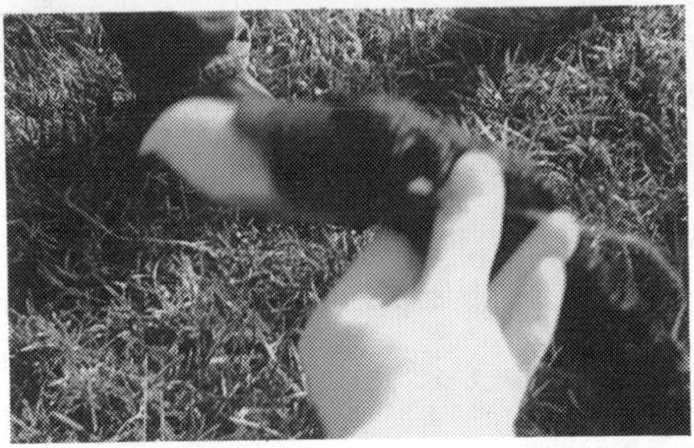

The Newborn Foal

The legs and hooves of a newborn are much different than an adult donkey. Newborn donkey foals have very pointed hooves. They are also very sharp around the edges and a swift kick, which newborns love to do, can cause a serious cut to the owner who is laying on the ground, ooohing and aaahing this adorable baby.

All foals are born with soft pads covering the hooves which protect the jennet's reproductive tract during late gestation and while giving birth. In the equine they are known an "golden slippers".

The frog of the hoof also has "frog feathers". They are also padding over the frog of the hoof to add additional padding and protection to the soft tender frog just after birth. As the baby makes his attempts to stand, these feathers soon dry and shrivel up. Both frog feathers and the golden slippers are normally worn off within 12 hours if the foal is walking on dirt however it may take longer if the foal is in a stall heavily bedded with soft straw bedding.

Some foals are born with weak flexor tendons or lax ligaments. This "down at the pastern" appearance puts the fetlocks closer to the ground and in some cases, touching the ground. Most ligaments tighten up with age and activity and you can see a noticeable difference in two to three days however, other cases may take three or four weeks or even months to straighten.

When examining a foal's legs, remember that they generally stand differently than they walk. Therefore, it is extremely important to watch a foal in motion. Most young foals stand toed-out for balance yet walk perfectly straight. Think about yourself when you are having a casual conversation while standing. Most likely, your legs are spread apart more for balance, than they are when you are walking.

Viewing the legs

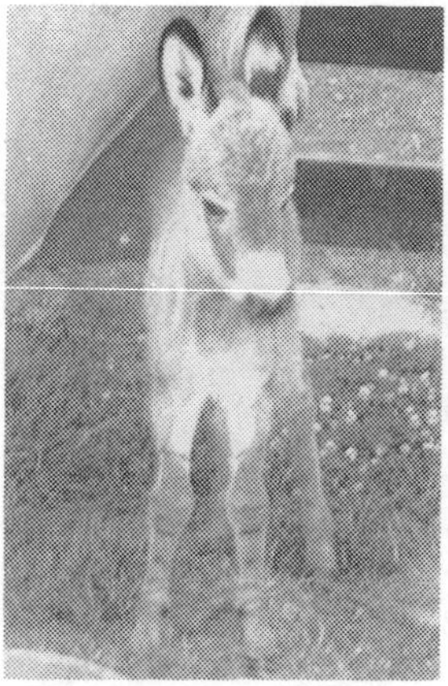

The newborn is standing toed-out for balance

Legs should be viewed from three different angles: from directly in front, from the side and from the top of the shoulder looking down. Make certain that the donkey is standing on perfectly level ground.

Stand directly in front of the foal. Take a yardstick and with the thinnest side facing you, hold it in the middle of the upper forearm and hold it straight down. The yardstick should fall in the middle of the forearm, knee, cannon and hoof.

You will notice that most foals have some deviation at the knees showing slight knock-knees. This deviation should be <u>mild</u>. Kneel down and watch the foal walk toward you. He

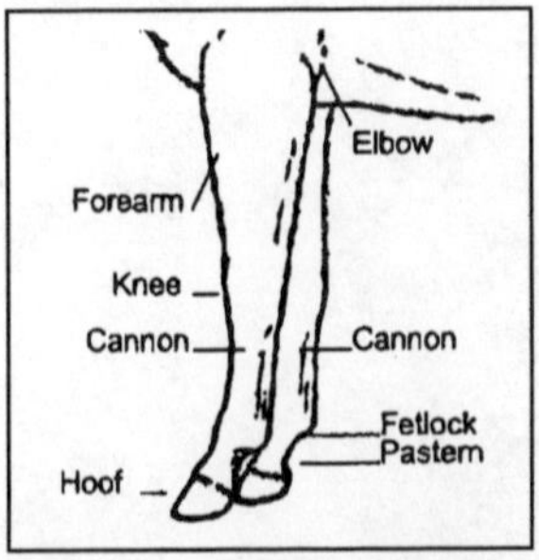

should not paddle out when he walks.

After viewing many many Miniature Donkeys, I have noticed a serious conformation flaw being passed along, unknowingly by breeders. Most people have been educated through the pages of **MDT**, and are aware of the problem with cowhocks and donkeys. However, few people are knowledgeable about a problem with crooked front legs - toed-out or knock knees. These two conformation flaws are easily passed on to foals. No jack with abnormal toed-out front legs or knock knees should ever be used as a herd sire.

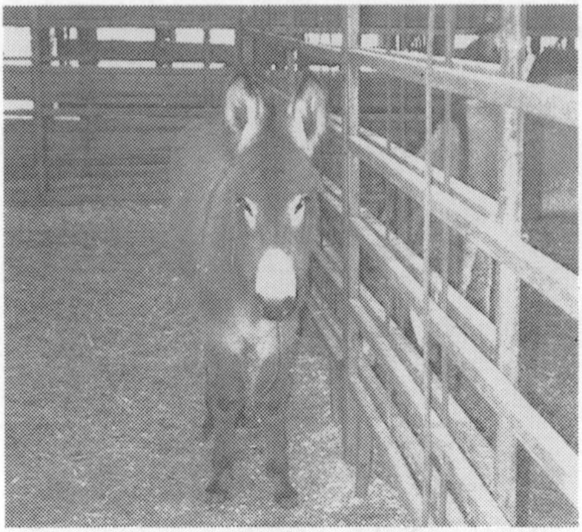

This youngster is both knock-kneed and severely toed-out

On the other hand, there are straight legged jacks who can remove this flaw from the legs of foals out of mildly crooked-legged jennets. This is another reason why you should be very critical of your herd sire or a jack you are considering purchasing as a herd sire. This also allows you to buy less-than-perfect jennets.

Side View, front legs:

You can do the same with the side view as you would with the front view. Drop a yardstick from the middle of the top of the forearm straight down. It should bisect the middle of the knee and the yardstick should end directly behind the back of the hoof. The cannon should always be longer than the forearm.

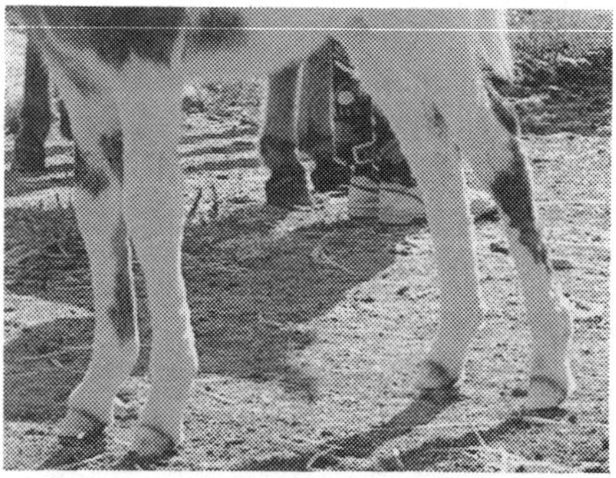

This foal clearly shows a too short forearm and a too long cannon

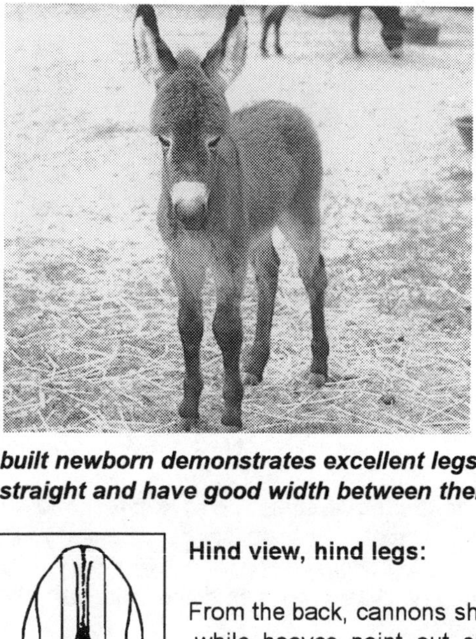

This finer built newborn demonstrates excellent legs. All four are straight and have good width between them.

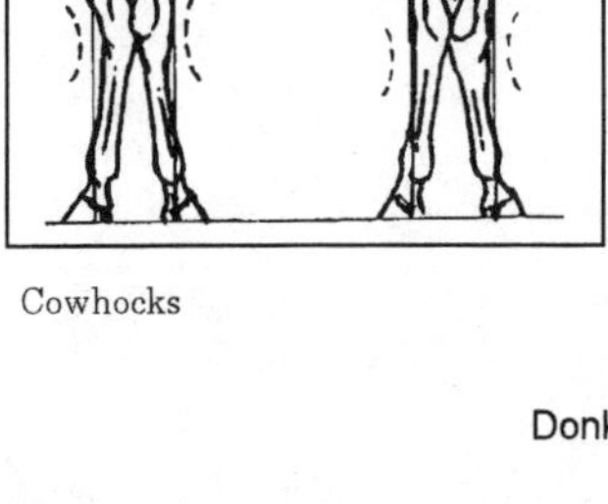

Cowhocks

Hind view, hind legs:

From the back, cannons should be parallel, while hooves point out slightly to match the angle of the stifle joints.
Unlike the front hooves, it is normal for the hind hooves to point slightly outward. Back knees should not be touching, or even close to it, and if they are, your donkey is cow-hocked. Again, watch the foal as it walks away from you and observe him at several different view points. Many times

foals - and adults - stand cow-hocked while relaxed, however this does not mean that the animal is cow-hocked.

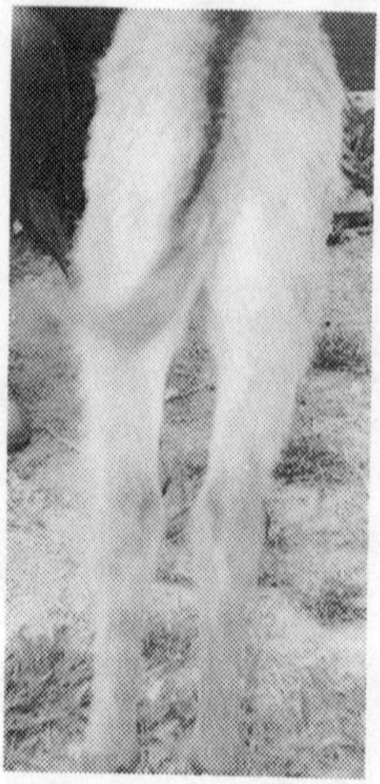

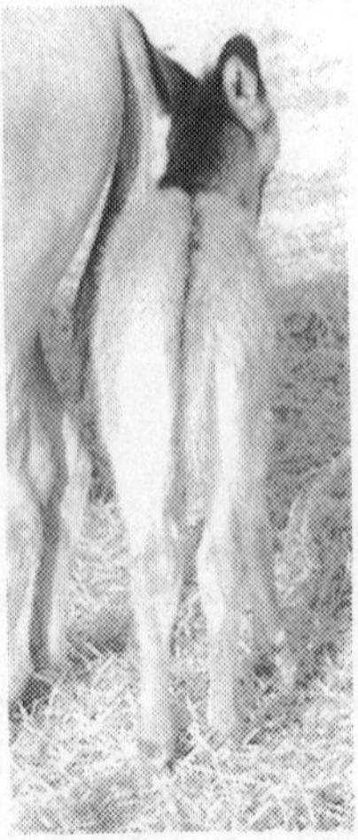

Newborns with nice straight legs

Maintaining Normal Legs and Feet

The hooves of donkeys under one year grow about twice as fast as adult donkeys. The back hooves on young donkeys grow very pointed. Long crooked hooves can and does cause permanent leg deformities. Most donkey foals, by the age of 6 weeks, need some type of hoof care and trimming. Foal hooves should be evaluated thereafter every four to six weeks.

If the foal needs corrective trimming, to help with crooked legs or hooves, they should be reevaluated every three weeks. Many farriers have no experience in trimming donkey hooves and either trim them too short, too long or cut off the heels like they would a horse. Our book, "*Caring For Your Miniature Donkey*" has a whole chapter on the proper way to trim donkey hooves along with numerous step-by-step pictures. Don't be shy about giving a copy to your farrier! They will in all probability be very thankful for the guidelines to follow.

What happens to the legs affects the hooves and what happens to the hooves affects the legs. Knowing what is normal for your donkey is just as important as knowing what is not. If you are not sure whether you have a

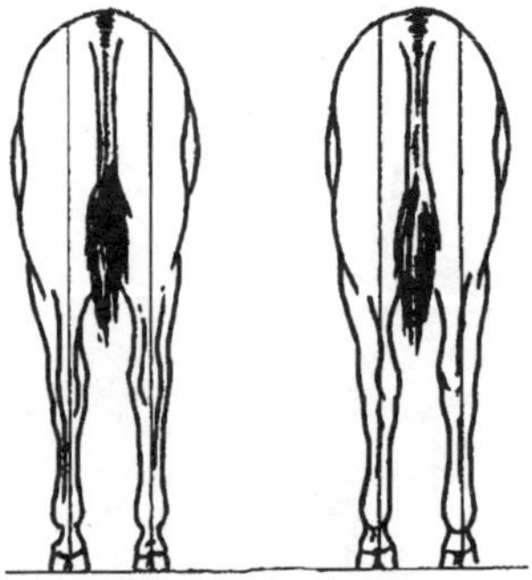

Left show very nice straight legs. Right shows slightly turned out at hock which is acceptable in donkeys

leg or hoof problem, call your veterinarian and let them examine the leg and hoof. It's better to have them say "that's normal, they'll grow out of it" then to let a problem persist and cause permanent damage.

Foal Hooves

Front hooves on donkey foals tend to grow very upright and if left to grow, your foal looks and feels like it is walking on stilts. Back hooves tend to grow very pointed and long in the toe. This ends up making the foal walk on its heels and is very hard on their tendons and ligaments. Your foal will become sickle hocked and cowhocked because of these long hooves. The only way they can walk is toed out or cowhocked because they cannot break over the front of the hoof like they should. During this most important time when the foal's bones are forming, if you do not correct this, it will come a permanent defect.

Hemolytic Disease

Hemolytic disease is a severe red blood cell destroying disease of newborn foals. It can ONLY occur when a foal and its SIRE possess a blood factor ABSENT in the jennet. During pregnancy, some of the foal's blood may pass into the jennet's circulation. If the foal has inherited a blood type that is different from the jennet, her blood will treat the foal's red blood cells as foreign bodies.

Antibodies - produced by the jennet - to fight these are stored in the jennet's first milk. When the foal receives the colostrum, the antibodies absorbed through the intestine begin to attack and destroy his red blood cells. The jennet can be "sensitized" by their foal if some placental disease allows the passage of blood from the foal to the dam. Normally, this does not occur, which is why the foal is not affected when it is born.

These foals are quite healthy when they are born and nurse normally. Within 12 to 36 hours, they become dull, weak, do not nurse and they may collapse. Mucous membranes may be pale for the first 24 hours, developing jaundice (yellowing) within 24 to 48 hours that gets progressively worse. Death may occur from acute anemia within 12 to 36 hours. Frequently, foals survive only three or four days.

Most antibodies are removed from the jennet's milk within 8 to 16 hours, IF she is milked by hand every hour. After 48 to 72 hours, it is usually safe to return a foal to the jennet. In jennets who have an immune response, they may be safely bred ONLY to jacks whose blood is compatible with their own.

White Muscle Disease

White Muscle Disease occurs when there is an inadequate dietary intake of selenium and vitamin E, and severely affects the muscles of the animal. Vitamin E and selenium function jointly to protect and stabilize cell membranes, including muscle cell membranes. Vitamin E serves as the "first line" oxidant, which decreases peroxide formation by the tissues. Excessive peroxides are destroyed by the selenium-containing tissue enzyme.

Vitamin E and selenium [work together] in effect stabilizing cell membranes and therefore both are generally believed to play a part in the [production and development] of white muscle disease. The independent and joint roles of vitamin E and selenium in this disease have been established in other species. Controversy over these roles in horses still exists. Selenium administered alone (without vitamin E) seems to be effective in both treatment and prevention of white muscle disease. This finding suggests that, in field situations, inadequate dietary intake of selenium may be more important than inadequate vitamin E intake in the development of the disease.

White muscle disease occurs primarily in areas of the United States and Canada that have selenium deficient soil, **which in turn results in selenium deficient grains and forage**.

This article summarizes the histories and clinical signs of 11 foals with white muscle disease that were presented to the Large Animal Clinic at the

New York State College of Veterinary Medicine, Cornell University. Autopsy findings of 6 of the 11 foals that died in the large animal clinic and 4 foals that were sent in after death from the surrounding area are also given.

History and Clinical Signs

The foals affected with white muscle disease were from New York, Pennsylvania and Maine, which are known to be states with selenium-deficient soil. Mares of affected foals and foals old enough to eat solid food were on diets composed of locally grown crops. The incidence of the diseases was not apparently breed or sex-related in these foals. *(Ed Note: There is documentation of Miniature Donkey foals dying and Miniature Donkey jennets aborting due to white muscle disease.)* Onset of signs in 14 of the foals varied from birth to 11 months of age; five foals were affected at birth, one at 7 hours of age, one at 4 days of age, four between 2 and 8 weeks of age, and three between 4 and 11 months of age. **One fetus with histologic [tissue] lesions of white muscle disease was aborted at 10 months gestation.** One foal (11 months old) was affected after its first period of exercise following a winter of confinement. The disease had a seasonal incidence corresponding to the foaling season; 13 of the total 15 foals studied became ill between February and June. The

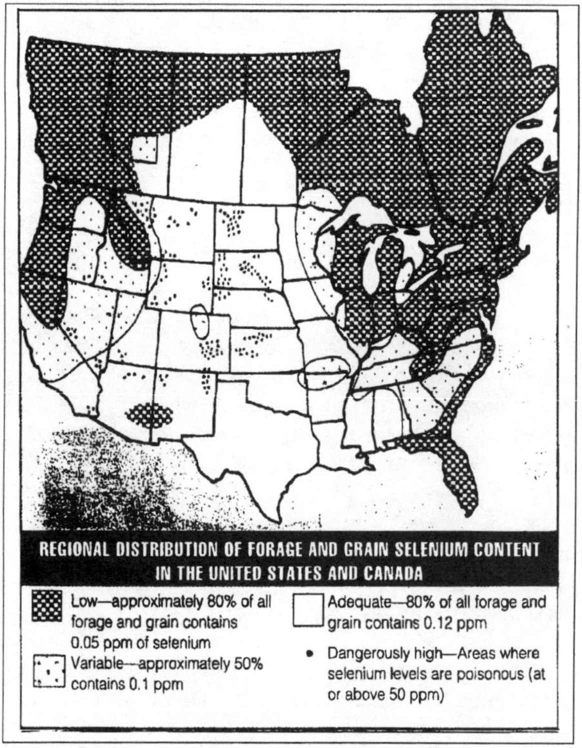

11 foals presented to the Large Animal Clinic initially were bright and alert. Depression was only apparent in the terminal state of the disease. Rectal temperatures were recorded in 10 foals and ranged from 97 to 104 degrees. Three of the 10 foals had temperatures higher than 101.5 degrees. Of these three foals, one had [existing blood poisoning], one had pneumonia and the third had excessive muscular activity (thrashing attributed to unsuccessful attempts to stand) that was thought to have caused the [fever].

Muscle [malfunction] was apparent on physical examination in all 11 cases. The clinical signs varied, depending on distribution of muscular lesions. Weakness was present in 10 of 11 foals. The one foal that was not weak presented [difficulty in swallowing] as its only abnormality. Eight foals were unable to rise without assistance; the muscles of the chest and/or pelvic limbs were affected in these foals. A few of the eight foals made active attempts to rise but would violently fall and roll, which was occasionally misinterpreted as colic. In 5 of the 11 foals presented, a stiff, painful gait was observed; tense painful muscles were palpable in 4 foals. [Difficulty in swallowing] was evident in 7 of 11 foals as oral or nasal regurgitation of milk after nursing. Two foals were unable to nurse because of pain associated with extending the neck. All foals had an elevated respiratory rate. Three foals had [difficulty in breathing], two of these had [bluish] mucous membranes.

Clinical data

Urine was a coffee-brown color grossly in three of the seven patients from which urine was obtained. Protein and blood were reported in all of the urinalyses except one foal.

Treatment

Physical exertion of the foals was minimized to avoid further muscle damage. Vitamin E-selenium (E-SE7 - Schering) was administered by intramuscular injection at a dose of 1 ml/45 kg of body weight. This was repeated in the surviving foals at 3 days and again at 8 to 10 days after the initial injection. Foals that exhibited [difficulty in swallowing] were given milk and oral electrolytes by nasal tube. Severely dehydrated foals were treated with intravenous fluids.

Anti-inflammatory drugs were administered to help reduce muscle pain and swelling. Because these drugs can cause ulcers in foals, they were only administered for two days. Foals were put in well-bedded environments with good footing to minimize further muscle trauma associated with efforts to rise.

Postmortem Findings

Six of the 11 foals admitted to the Large Animal Clinic had advanced signs, failed to respond to therapy, and died. [Autopsy] findings confirmed muscle degeneration in all cases. The location of the affected muscles varied but correlated well with the clinical signs displayed by each foal. Affected muscles included those of the thoracic limbs, pelvic limbs, and heart; cervical muscles; the diaphragm and the tongue. [Lesions of the heart muscle] were evident in 5 of the 10 foals autopsied **including a fetus that had been aborted at 10 months gestation**. Aspiration pneumonia was apparent in two foals.

Conclusions

The clinical diagnosis of white muscle disease is based on a combination of clinical signs showing muscle disease, elevated enzymes in muscle, decreased blood selenium and response to vitamin E-selenium administration. [Observation] evaluation is more important than laboratory evaluation in arriving at an accurate prognosis. Foals where appropriate therapy is delayed have a very poor prognosis. *(Ed Note: Unfortunately, in the case of tiny miniature donkey foals, by the time a diagnosis is made, it is usually too late for treatment to be effective. The best treatment is* ***prevention*** *discussed later in this report.)* Foals that are unable to support weight with assistance have a poor prognosis, as do foals with dark brown urine. Unfortunately, definitive diagnosis requires autopsy or biopsy. Relative assurance of a clinical diagnosis of white muscle disease, elevation of muscle enzymes, and decreased blood selenium.

If a diagnosis of white muscle disease is suspected, blood selenium values should be determined in the sick foal as well as in other foals and jennets on the same farm to assess the selenium status of the herd. *(Ed Note: In an interview with Dr. Hintz of Cornell, we were advised that if a foal is diagnosed with white muscle disease, all future foals out of that same mother should be put on an immediate prevention program. She should be fed selenium supplemented feed and blood evaluations should be done on her every 3 months to monitor blood selenium levels.)* Evaluation of the herd is important because mild selenium deficiencies may result in decreased immune response to infectious diseases in foals.

Prevention

White muscle disease can be prevented in foals by injecting selenium and vitamin E at birth and by selenium supplementation of pregnant jennets. Feed should be supplemented with selenium at 0.1 to 0.2 ppm [parts per million]. *(Ed Note: USDA has recently approved a .03 ppm additive to grain. Selenium is extremely toxic so you must first do several things. You must first determine the deficiency of selenium* ***in your area****. This can be done by (1) having your soil tested and (2) drawing blood from several donkeys in your herd and having selenium evaluation done. This will tell your feed dealer whether he needs to add 0.1, 0.2 or 0.3 ppm to your feed. Everyone in selenium deficient areas should have selenium added to the* *grain they feed their donkeys, however the question remains as to how much is to be added.)*

Although the FDA has approved maximal selenium supplementation at 0.3 mb/kg of dry matter in complete feeds for cattle, sheep, and swine, selenium supplementation of EQUINE feeds is restricted only by nutritional recommendations and industry practices. The selenium requirement of the horse was estimated at 0.1 mg/kg of diet. It was concluded that there was no advantage in supplementing the mature idle horse with more than 0.1 mg of selenium to prevent problems associated with selenium deficiency. (Ed Note: In the above mentioned interview with Dr. Hintz of Cornell, we were advised that a premixed feed with 0.1 mg.kg of selenium (feed 1-1/2 lbs of grain per day per donkey) was adequate in all areas EXCEPT the states of Oregon and Washington which need supplementation of 0.3 mg/kg mixed in feed.)

Selenium supplementation of pregnant jennets should be started six to eight weeks [before birth] in jennets found to be at risk. **Important Note: Only limited amounts of inorganic selenium cross the placenta, but organic selenium appears to cross the placenta more readily.** *(Ed Note: What this means is in areas of the country where natural selenium is in the grass and hay, enough passes through the placenta to protect the foal. Inorganic selenium would be selenium that is injected into the jennet before she foals, which this report indicates is NOT sufficient as not enough of it crosses the placenta.)*

A foal's blood selenium levels at birth are about one half of the blood selenium levels of its supplemented dam. Foals considered to be at risk should be treated at birth with 1 cc E-SE per 100 pounds of body weight (average would be 2/10ths of one cc of E-SE) administered intramuscularly. This could be repeated at approximately two and six weeks of age in an at-risk foal. *(Ed Note: Because this is a toxic substance, donkey foals must be weighed and treated with the exact amount. THERE ARE 3 DIFFERENT TYPES OF INJECTABLE SELENIUM!!! The three different names are "BO-SE", "MU-SE", and "ESE". All three have different dosages. The "ESE" is specifically made for equine, however, I am told that in areas heavily populated with cattle, some vets give the "MU-SE" (made for cattle) to equine. I have not yet heard of any bad effects however, I would recommend you have your vet give you the "ESE" for your donkeys. If giving BO-SE to a miniature donkey, give 5/10ths of one cc.*

Jennets on selenium supplementation have a higher milk selenium content than jennets not on supplementation, BUT selenium is not concentrated in the milk in sufficient quantities to protect the foals

from developing white muscle disease. Therefore, pre-injecting pregnant jennets before foaling is not a solution. Some controversy exists as to the usefulness of vitamin E in commercially available injectable vitamin E-selenium preparations. The amount of vitamin E provided at the recommended dose is not generally a sufficient quantity to be of value to a foal. Some question also exists as to how well vitamin E is absorbed when given intramuscularly. As mentioned previously, the precise roles of vitamin E and selenium in contributing to the onset of white muscle disease remain to be determined. Despite these controversies, parenteral treatment includes the provision of both selenium and vitamin E. Vitamin E and selenium interact to protect and stabilize cell membranes, including the muscle cell membrane. Selenium may enhance vitamin E uptake and storage.

(Ed Note: Since selenium deficiency is directly related to muscle inadequacies, SE-E deficiencies could also tie in with fixation of the patella in older donkeys. Strong leg muscles are needed to hold the patella in place. If your donkeys lack adequate muscle tone, you may want to consider selenium deficiency as the culprit.)

On the other hand......

Selenium intoxication

Selenium intoxication can result from excessive supplementation with selenium compounds. Toxicosis can also occur where the selenium content of the soil is high. Soils that contain more than 0.5 ppm of selenium are considered potentially dangerous. Seleniferous soils are found in the Great Plains south to Texas and Mexico, west to California, and east to Alabama in the United States and the prairie provinces of Canada.

The toxicity of selenium depends on the chemical form of selenium ingested, the duration of intake, and other components of the diet. Organic selenium compounds found in plants are most toxic. Acute selenium intoxication occurs in animals accidentally given excessive amounts of selenium compounds and in animals that rapidly consume large amounts in plants. Acute toxicity results in respiratory distress, diarrhea, prostration and death. A single oral dose of 3.3 mg of selenium per kilogram of body weight can be lethal to horses. Subacute or chronic selenium poisoning, also called "alkali disease", occurs when livestock consume feeds containing 5 to 40 ppm of selenium. Excess selenium can build up in the equine over a period of time causing various symptoms of hoof degeneration, lameness cirrhosis of the liver and others. Affected equine are often emaciated and lame and as the condition progresses, the hoof separates at the coronary band. Loss of mane and tail hair is often seen.

White Muscle Disease occurs in newborn foals up to the age of seven months and is a result of selenium deficient pastures. It is quite common in several states.

Chapter 8

Weanlings

Baby Boosters

Vaccinating foals is important, but when should you do it and what should you give?

Foals, just as infants, are vulnerable to disease and infection because their young bodies are naive to the world of germs and bacteria, which can cause those problems. So the inclination, particularly for equine owners who choose to vaccinate their own animals, is to administer vaccines as early as possible or as recommended by over-the-counter products. New research, however, seems to indicate that doing so may be a moot point in the very young.

Currently, the majority of vaccines offer only limited protection for the highly susceptible equine neonate, and therefore, attention should be given to decreasing exposure to pathogens, or those organisms which can cause disease, through isolation and sanitation, as well as by eliminating stressors that reduce the foal's resistance.

Factors that effect a foal immunization program include the management situation, geographic location and risk versus cost benefits for the owner. Although it is impossible to make universal recommendations for the vaccination of foals, a rational plan can be developed if the key decision points in passive or active immunization regimes are understood.

Nature's vaccination

Passive immunity is best understood as the immunity transferred to the foal by its mother through the colostrum the foal ingests as it first suckles. It is critical the. foal receive this colostrum, which is loaded with maternal antibodies, within the first few hours of life.

The value of passive immunity can be considerably influenced by vaccination of the mare in order to maximize the concentration of the antibodies present in the colostrum. All mares should receive booster vaccinations four to six weeks before giving birth using only killed (inactivated) agents. Typically, this includes vaccinations for tetanus, encephalomyelitis viruses, influenza and rhinopneumonitis, with additional vaccines for Streptococcus equi, Potomac Horse Fever, and in some circumstances, botulism. In previously unvaccinated mares, an initial vaccination course should be administered with the last booster given four to six weeks before foaling.

It Is also important to remember that the value of colostral transfer of passive immunity can also be considerably increased if the mare is housed on the farm where she is going to foal for six to eight weeks before foaling. This allows adequate time for the generation of immune responses to pathogens present on the farm and subsequent transfer of these antibodies into the colostrum. One general rule is that modified live vaccines (MLVs) are not given during pregnancy. Remember that an MLV will induce some type of infection itself in order to achieve immunization.

Passive immunization is also achieved by the oral administration of immunoglobin-containing products to foals in the first hours of life or by injection at any time. It is relatively common practice to administer tetanus antitoxin to neonatal foals. However, this provides relatively short-lived protection and carries the risk of inducing serum sickness in the foal. This policy is unnecessary if the mare is appropriately vaccinated during pregnancy.

For those foals who do not receive immunity through passive transfer, the administration of plasma transfusions is a common procedure and offers an opportunity to influence resistance to specific pathogens through the choice of product. Commercial equine plasma products should be chosen that have been prepared from donors extensively vaccinated against common equine pathogens.

Timing

A contentious issue in foal vaccination Is the timing of the initial series of vaccinations. The problem largely results from the effects of maternal antibodies received through the colostrum and their variable half life. It is difficult to time these initial vaccinations in the foal so that it is effective and administered early enough so as not to leave the young animal unprotected after the waning of material antibodies. An additional consideration is the increasing perception that foals may be relatively immunologically unresponsive to many of the currently available vaccines.

The first step in determining when to start a foal vaccination regime is knowing the duration of maternally derived antibodies. The rate of decline of maternal antibodies varies for both individuals and different infectious agents. For many important pathogens, the concentration of maternal antibodies in foals falls to nonprotective levels by two to three months of age. However, the remaining antibody, which one could view as residual, can still render the foal unresponsive to vaccination for weeks or even months to come.

Because, in the case of equine influenza, maternal antibodies can persist until six months of age and prevent immune responses in foals younger than six months. American Association of Equine Practitioners recommends beginning foal vaccinations at three to four months of age, followed by boosters at four week intervals. This is adequate for many foals, but a significant number are in a high-risk situation and may remain vulnerable to infection.

A more intensive vaccination schedule would include an initial vaccination at two months of age and monthly boosters until six months of age, with further boosters at nine and 12 months. In the case of tetanus and rabies, an initial vaccination at three to four months and a booster for weeks later should be adequate.

Even when intense vaccination regimes are used in young foals, poor responses can still be observed. This may be a result of a relative lack of immune responsiveness in young foals to currently available vaccines, but an alternative proposal is that the frequent use of vaccines in the face of persistent maternal immunity may actually induce a state of tolerance, which can prevent a satisfactory response to vaccines past one year of age.

What to use

Currently available vaccines include many highly effective products that are safe, provide long-term immunity and are practical to use. In making choices between products, one must consider both the antigen contained in the vaccine and the means of delivery. For example, in the case of equine influenza vaccines, it is important to look for an equine influenza type 2 strain with a date from the late 1980s or ideally the 1990s. This will increase the likelihood that the vaccine will protect against currently circulating strains of influenza virus. Similarly in the case of Equine Herpes Virus vaccines, it is important to include both EHV-1 and EHV-4 antigens for protection against both abortion and respiratory disease.

Most importantly, however, equine owners need to be aware that immunities develop based on exposure and protection. With the help of your veterinarian, you should be able to determine the appropriate vaccination schedule best for your animals, both young and old.

References: AAEP - Reprinted by permission. D. Paul Lunn, BV5C, PhD, MRCVS, Dipi. ACVIM

Weaning Strategies

Minimizing the stress levels means a healthier foal -- and fewer frazzled nerves for you!

No one looks forward to weaning time. There's nothing quite as heart-rending as the sound of a panicky foal, galloping and up and down the fence-line and calling desperately for the mother who's been taken away -- **unless** it's the sound of his dam, calling back! It's no wonder so many owners dread this duty; it pushes the guilt buttons like nothing else.

Still, we know that weaning is a necessary part of the process of growing up for a foal. It's also important for the jennet's well-being, particularly if she has been bred back and is carrying next year's foal, because nursing makes significant demands on her nutritional resources and may leave her looking like a hat-rack. Wrenching though it may be, it's got to be done. The question, then, is how to make weaning as painless as possible.

Researchers describe an animal as in a state of stress if it must make abnormal or extreme changes in its physiology or behavior to cope with the adverse effects of its environment or management. Under that definition, weaning definitely qualifies as a source of stress to youngsters of many species. Minimizing stress during the weaning process is more than a matter of peace of mind (or peace and quiet). Studies have demonstrated that foals who suffer undue stress when being weaned may lose their appetites and lose weight -- and then later, when they recover, they often undergo a sudden growth spurt. The result of this dip and surge in the growth curve of a young equine is sometimes a case of developmental orthopedic disease (DOD), the condition in which bones and joints begin to develop abnormally, causing contracted tendons, physitis, or even bone cysts in the joints of the limbs. In contrast, foals who undergo the minimum amount of stress during weaning continue to grow on a more even keel (their heights and weights increase in smooth increments). And that, researchers say, makes them far less predisposed to DOD.

In addition, stressed foals are prone to gastric ulcers (which can further delay their growth and development), delayed reproductive function, and a host of opportunistic bacterial and viral infections, such as strangles, influenza, equine herpes virus (formerly known as rhinopneumonitis), and salmonella. This is because under stress, equine experience increased levels of cortisol, a hormone secreted by the adrenal cortex, in their bloodstreams. In the short term, a raised cortisol level is a good thing -- it assists the "fight or flight" response that helps keep equine alive in times of crisis. But when the cortisol level remains high for long periods of time (as it often does during weaning), the hormone can compromise a foal's

normal immune function and leave him vulnerable to disease.
A stressed foal doesn't sleep well. Foals in general need more sleep than do adult donkeys, and to sleep soundly, they must be in laternal recumbency (stretched out on the ground, not lying on their sternums). Researchers have suggested that the release of hormones, especially the all-important (to foals) growth hormone, and the process of cell division, are intricately related to the sleep cycle -- so in a very real sense, a stressful weaning may stunt a foal's growth.

Finally, because an anxious foal is often a panicky one, undue stress during weaning can increase the likelihood of injuries -- either from running up and down the fence-line till immature joints are overloaded, or by tangles with fence-lines or with other donkeys. For all of these reasons, then, it's in the best interests of the foal (and by extension, his owner) to de-stress the weaning process as much as possible.

Weaning: When Is He Ready?

Opinions vary as to when is the best time to wean foals, but most breeding farm managers aim for somewhere in the range of four to six months of age. Ideally, three things should be in place before a foal is ready to wean:

- He should be sufficiently socialized with other donkeys that he will be able to behave himself in a herd without having mother there to intervene on his behalf. This behavior is usually established early on in foals who are raised in large groups, but may be delayed in foals who are raised as 'single' babies or who reside on small farms. It's a good idea to make sure the foal has been introduced to a 'substitute companion' -- a patient older gelding, barren jennet, or another donkey -- who can serve as both a friendly face, and in some cases, as a disciplinarian, to a foal about to be weaned.

- He should be nutritionally independent -- that is, he should not be deriving most of his nourishment from his dam's milk. Early in a foal's life, milk is his only food, but even from the age of a couple of weeks, he begins to show interest in the grass, hay, and grain his mother eats. From that initial curious sampling, he should progress to regular consumption of a creep ration, so that by the age of four months or so, he is deriving most of his nutritional needs from solid food, and only returns to the 'dairy bar' (which by now, is producing much less milk) on an occasional basis and more for comfort than anything else.

- This brings us to the third requirement of a ready-to-be-weaned foal: emotional independence. A young foal is initially a shadow of his dam -- tagging along very close to her side, and too frightened of the world and all its confusing inhabitants to stray very far. But with each passing day, a foal's curiosity gradually overcomes his fear, and his dependency on Mom diminishes as he becomes bold enough to venture forth and explore his environment. Some are naturally more gregarious than others, of course, so this may happen at different rates, but a foal who is ready to be weaned is one who already spends a good deal of his time away from his mother's side. A younger foal, still emotionally dependent, would likely be far more traumatized by his dam's sudden absence than an older, braver one.

These, of course, are the preferred conditions. But under certain circumstances -- such as the illness, injury, or death of the jennet -- it is sometimes necessary to wean a foal younger than four months of age. If you find yourself in this awkward position, recognize that the weaning process is likely to be very hard on your foal, and be prepared to provide nutritional support (in the form of milk replacers if he is too young for solid rations) as well as emotional aid (both through increased human contact, and possibly by providing him with a nurse jennet or babysitter, such as a patient pony).

Before you wean your foal, you should accustom him to the stall and/or paddock where he will be weaned, so that he thoroughly knows the layout and will be less likely to hurt himself. It goes without saying that the area you use should be triple-checked for safety. There should be no protruding nails or sharp edges anywhere; hardware, such as buckets and hangers, should be kept to a minimum, and fencing should be high enough to discourage a foal from trying to leap over it, and able to take the impact of his anguished little body without shattering or giving way. Many farms consider tight 'diamond' wire mesh, topped with oak rails, to be the safest arrangement, but board fencing, while not particularly forgiving, can be solid enough to discourage shenanigans and is also a popular choice. Page wire, however, with its large, open weave, is a dangerous fence for volatile weanlings, and any fence of low visibility, such as some types of high-tensile wire, is also a bad idea.

Before you forge ahead, put together a game plan for weaning. Many farm managers feel that weaning is stressful enough for a foal without introducing him to new surroundings and new companions at the same time -- so on the whole, it's usually easier to remove the jennet to another location, than it is to move the foal. While jennets do also suffer stress as a result of the weaning process (as indicated by their raised cortisol levels, which usually persist for about 24 hours post-separation from their offspring), their greater maturity means they adapt sooner, particularly in the case of 'career' broodmares who have been through it many times before.

Whether you remove the jennet to another farm entirely, or just to a location out of earshot of her foal, is a matter of convenience; but whichever you choose, you must keep in mind that it will take her a few days to 'dry up' (stop producing milk). During those few days, she is likely to be sore and disagreeable, but resist the temptation to milk her out to relieve her discomfort; by stimulating the glands, you only perpetuate the milk production. Many farm managers find that reducing the jennet's grain ration (or eliminating it completely) for a few days assists in the drying out process.

Do you intend to wean your foal in a paddock situation, or in a stall? This will depend on your facilities, and you should choose whichever environment is likely to be safer for your new weanling during that initial frantic phase when panic first sets in. It's more difficult to control a foal who is loose in a paddock -- but if he is in a group situation, perhaps with a 'baby-sitter' gelding or older jennet, he may exhibit fewer signs of stress in that environment. Truth be told, some foals fail to register that their dams have disappeared at first, when they are engaged in group play with other foals in their herd. On the other hand, keeping your foal in a stall means you have better access to him should he need attention (or just human comfort), and the confinement probably reduces the overall risk of injury. If you intend to have more than one foal in a stall or paddock, remember that an upset foal can sometimes become violent -- so provide sufficient room for each to stay out of the other's way!

The period of time immediately pre- or post-weaning is not the time to vaccinate or de-worm your foal, get his hooves trimmed, or teach him to lead or tie. Not only is the foal likely to be distracted and thus very uncooperative, but any one of these demands could act as a stress multiplier, the last thing he needs. Ideally, vaccinations, de-worming, and basic halter-breaking should have been done some time before weaning; if not, wait at least a couple of weeks after your foal has been weaned to undertake them.

GOING COLD TURKEY

The $64,000 question when it comes to weaning is -- is it best to suddenly and completely separate mare/jennet and foal, or is it kinder to part them gradually?

According to a doctoral study by Cynthia McCall, Ph.D., at Texas A & M University in the 1980's, it appears that foals who had fence-line contact with their dams during the first week of weaning showed greatly reduced signs of stress (vocalizations, fretfulness, and adrenal cortisol levels in the bloodstream) when compared to foals separated abruptly from their mothers. In fact, their behavioral and physiological responses to weaning weren't significantly different than those exhibited by foals who were not weaned at all. The fence-line method allowed mares and foals to see, touch, and smell each other, but prevented nursing. McCall suspects that not only does this method of gradual weaning reduce foal anxiety, it may also, in the end, reduce the incidence of injuries ... and because serum cortisol levels were not as elevated, the immune response in foals weaned this way may not be as severely compromised, meaning less risk of post-weaning illness. McCall notes, "I think the gradual approach is easier on everyone. After a while the mares just wander off, and everyone's happy."

(MDT Ed Note: I really found this study interesting as here at Pheasant Meadow Farm we have found the exact opposite to be true! Just two years ago we had a group of 5 weanlings that we were keeping. We put them in a pasture that borders the pasture where their mothers were. For weeks on end, the dams thought of nothing but standing on the opposite side of the fence or running the fence line braying, even going so far as neglecting to eat or drink. It drove the mothers, foals and me bonkers! This demonstrates the difference in how donkeys and horses act to the same situation. We've found the 'ol out of sight, out of mind practice to be best to be much more suitable for donkeys where dams can neither see nor hear their weanlings. The weanlings do great and the dams give up their search within 24 hours and rejoin the herd.)

However, there are some physiological indications that gradual separation may just prolong the stress response in both mares/jennets and foals. The practice some farms use, of separating dams and foals during the day, and reuniting them at night (or vice versa) essentially jump-starts the stress cycle anew each morning, and may result in elevated cortisol levels -- and all their associated damaging effects -- which last for weeks. A single, final separation, then, might be best for all concerned.

"There's no doubt that the weaning process is a painful one," says Karyn Malinowski, Ph.D., of Rutgers University; "but it's a short-lived stress if you do it right. I prefer to cut the umbilical cord, so to speak, and get it over with, on the theory that acute short-term stress is probably less harmful than prolonging it and creating *chronic* stress. It's like quitting smoking, I think."

I WANT TO BE ALONE

Malinowski also notes that human contact may help to relieve stress in a fretful foal. In her study, many of the foals weaned by themselves were so agitated that they had to remain under close surveillance -- and human intervention was needed on more than one occasion. That contact and handling may have had a positive effect on the immune function of the singly weaned foals.

In fact, foals who are accustomed to being handled by humans are likely to suffer far less stress during the weaning process than those who have been left to run 'wild and woolly'. If your presence is seen as comforting, rather than something else to be alarmed about, the foal may very well relax and begin to accept you as a substitute authority figure -- which of course is exactly what you want to establish in your young horse's training. Consider yourself an active participant in the weaning process, even if it tears at your heartstrings at first to hear your foal's distress calls. The payoff will be a minimally painful weaning process, and with luck, a very-soon-well-adjusted young weanling ready to progress towards equine adulthood.

Reference: Written by Karen Briggs an accomplished horsewoman and writer.

Foal Nutrition, Deworming and Vaccinations

Nutrition: Most foals will begin to nibble on grass and hay at around one week of age. You can introduce your foal to grain at two to four weeks of age. Some people are under the impression that withholding grain and feeding low quality hay will help keep the donkey small. All this actually does is temporarily slow down its growth and could cause poor bone formation. Your foal will grow eventually to its intended height, however, may take longer to do so. Sufficient grain and good quality hay will help assure your foal's good health.

Worming and Immunization: Your foals first worming should be based on several factors. How many animals do you have per acre and how much manure your foal is subjected to. Your vet should be able to advise you, depending on your circumstances, when the first worming should be. A good rule of thumb would be at age 4 to 6 weeks and monthly thereafter until the age of 6 months. They would then be put on your regular worming schedule - every two months. It is important to note that unlike mature donkeys, foals frequently have infestations of strongyloides and ascarids. Therefore, the parasite control program for donkeys under one year of age should be effective against those parasites. Check the labels on your wormers. NOT ALL WORMERS ARE SAFE FOR FOALS. Make certain that whatever wormer you use has a statement from the manufacturer stating that it is safe to use on foals.

Foal Hoof Care

Foal hoof care is something most people tend to neglect. Most foals do a great deal of playing and running around, which helps keep their front hooves worn down and in fairly good shape. However, this is not the case regarding their back hooves. Donkey foal hooves become very pointed around the age of two months. Pointed hooves will not allow the foal to "break over" like they should when walking, but walk toed-out - cowhocked. This creates uneven stress on joints and stretches the adjacent ligaments during this most important time when your foal's bones are forming. Allowing your foal to continue in this cowhocked condition could cause permanent crooked limbs.

This problem is very easily solved with a blacksmith's rasp. Simply file off approximately 1/8" of the very tip of the toe, just enough to give the hoof a rounder affect similar to the front hooves.

Foals are still small enough at this age to handle by yourself. If you do have a foal who is a little too rambunctious for you to handle, have someone help you. Another person can help divert the foal's attention from you working on his hooves.

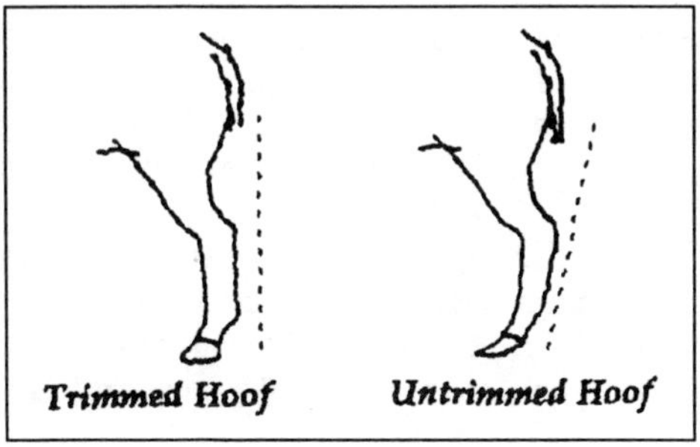

Reduce Risk to Foals During Winter

While the first 12 months of a foal's life are the most critical, much emphasis should be placed on the first six months of age. During this time, rapid growth is coupled with greater health risk than at any other time.

The first winter for weanlings is important due to their vulnerability. Consequently, winter management should aim toward minimizing stress and providing whatever is necessary to ensure the weanlings continue growing and remain healthy.

Housing and daily management are important considerations. In recent years, cost of production has changed how animals are managed. The number of weanlings, type of facilities and available labor determine how they will be handled daily. When there are several weanlings, they may be housed together. Usually, they are kept on pasture with a run-in shed for shelter.

It has been observed that most weanlings are healthier, with less respiratory problems, when kept on pasture with a run-in shed.

There is a consensus among many equine owners that weanlings that run outside are sounder than those kept in a stall most of the time during this stage of their life. Exercise has been observed to increase bone breaking strength, an indicator of strong bones.

Since weanlings are playful, there is the risk of more injuries when they are kept in groups. However, this is a trade off. There are few serious injuries and the weanlings are healthier, grow better and have sounder feet and legs when out.

It is usually no problem to have colts and fillies in the same group at this age.

Occasionally, a colt will be aggressive and attempt to mount fillies. He can be separated because of the potential injury from kicking and biting. There is not a problem from sexual contact until colts reach about 7 to 10 months of age and colts and fillies should be separated into two groups.

Weanlings are curious. Being active, they are more likely to have accidents. There should be adequate pasture area for each weanling. This is not to provide feedstuffs, since there is limited forage available during the winter months, as much as it is for adequate exercise. The area should not be too confining as weanlings like to run and play. The area should be rather long so foals can run with some speed or rather square so they can run in large circles. Another problem with small paddocks (or pastures) is they easily become muddy during bad weather. This increases the probability of injury as well as stress. There are many factors to be considered, however, at least one-fourth of an acre per weanling should be provided in group management. It is best to have several small pastures so the weanlings can be rotated from pasture to pasture. This will help keep the area from becoming muddy.

Fencing for weanlings is critical. It should be at least 5 feet high with a board at the top. The board should be 4 to 6 inches wide. Equine have poor eyesight and a board at the top will allow the weanlings to see the fence and prevent them from running into it.

Three-sided run-sheds provide protection from winter weather and a place for weanlings to eat and sleep. Weanlings like to stay closer together than older equine. The shed should be well bedded to encourage the weanlings to sleep inside, especially in inclement weather. Add bedding periodically to ensure dryness. This build-up of bedding inside the shed should be higher than the ground around the shed aiding in dryness and warmth. Wood shavings are a preferred bedding material for weanlings. Sawdust, if not too dusty, is also satisfactory especially in a run-in shed. Weanlings will tend to eat straw bedding.

Turning a weanling out by itself is risky with potential for injury. If possible, an individual weanling should be turned out with another donkey or horse for company, as well as to keep it calm. An older gelding or mare can be a good babysitter. It should be an animal with patience and one not likely to kick or bite the weanling. An older, quiet one can also help keep a group of weanlings calm. This procedure is especially helpful when they are first turned out together. Proper fencing for a single weanling is more critical than for several weanlings. The single weanling, if kept by itself in a paddock, is more likely to try and get to other donkeys and horses if it can see or hear them. With a single weanling, the owner can keep it in a stall at night and during inclement weather put out in a paddock during the day. This management procedure requires more labor but is usually not a problem for the one weanling owner.

Weanlings should have already been immunized for tetanus. Respiratory diseases are a problem with weanlings. Immunization against flu is recommended as is vaccination for Rhinopneumonitis. Rhinopneumonitis in young horses appears as a cough or "snots" while it causes abortion in broodmares. Donkey foals are usually immunized for flu and Rhinopneumonitis at [four to five] months of age. Booster shots are commonly given at 90 day intervals. It is important that weanlings to properly immunized against these respiratory threats.

Weanlings should also be on a regular deworming program every 30 to 60 days. A paste wormer is easy to administer to weanlings and results in little stress.

Nutrition is also significant during the winter. The growth rate of weanlings is less than that of sucklings, but it is still quite high. This level of growth requires considerable energy protein, minerals and vitamins. [Donkey weanlings can be fed free choice alfalfa/grass mixed hay.] It is advisable to have a hay rack in the run-in shed to keep rain and snow off the hay and provide a warm environment for the weanlings to eat. If the hay rack is outside, it should be situated on a high, dry area. Do not feed the hay on the floor of the run-in shed or on the ground. This greatly increases the reinfestation of parasites as well as wastes hay. Hay should be fed at a level of 1.5 pounds per 100 pounds of body-weight or free choice.

If a grass forage is fed to weanlings, a mineral mix of 8-12 percent calcium and 8-12 percent phosphorus should be fed. This level can be obtained with a mineral mix of one-half trace mineralized salt and one-half dicalcium phosphate. In addition, trace mineralized salt should be available.

Weanlings kept out during the winter will develop a heavy hair coat. They do not have to be groomed regularly, especially if they have a dry bedded area for sleep. Their feet should be given regular attention.

Reference: by Frederick Harper, Ph.D., Extension Animal Science-Horse, University of Tennessee

Winter Care of Weanlings

Most weanlings are between the age of six and nine months during the coldest part of winter. Their care is critical at this time as they are not only facing their first winter but are coming in contact with severe weather and potential health risks. Winter care should be aimed at minimizing stress to help them remain healthy. Hopefully you have not waited until the dead of winter before weaning your foal from its mother. If you had a late summer or early fall foal, and the mother is in good weight, you may have to keep the weanling with its mother until early spring if you are having a rough winter. You will have to pay extremely close attention to the mother to make very certain that she is not losing weight. With a winter coat, this means feeling her body along the back, rib cage and hips, not just looking, as long coats hide too much.

On most topics, you can ask 10 veterinarians one question and receive 10 different answers. When it concerns winter housing, you will probably only hear one answer. The more they are outside, the better and healthier that weanling will remain. You must also use common sense as we *are* talking about *miniatures.* Miniatures do not and cannot produce the amount of body heat that a full-grown horse can. If you live in Minnesota, the temperature is -10 with 30 mile an hour winds, that weanling needs to be inside a barn. We have fairly mild winters here in Maryland but do on occasion get snow and extreme temperatures. We have never had a problem with sickness during winter months as we follow several rules of thumb. Seldom are our donkeys locked inside a barn. Our barn doors remain open all year so the donkeys can come and go as they please. There are a few circumstances when we *will* lock the donkeys inside.
1. Expecting a snow storm at night. During the day, the barn remains open as we can keep an eye on things.
2. Freezing rain. The ground in front of our barn slopes down and can become very slippery.
3. Winds in excess of 20 miles per hour along with cold temperatures. Whether it be a barn or a run-in shed, donkeys cannot protect themselves from wind and winter coats alone are not enough protection.

Talk to any professional equine breeder or any veterinarian and they will tell you that airtight barns are a no-no even during severe winter temperatures. When raising donkeys or horses, you always have to keep the respiratory health of your animals in mind. Good respiratory health always means access to clean fresh air void of dust. If weather dictates that we need to stall weanlings due to inclement weather, we stall them together. Donkeys are very sociable animals so stalling separately would cause undue stress.

Weanlings are playful and need room to run and exercise. One half to one acre is plenty of room for five or six weanlings. If the paddock area is too small, they easily become muddy during bad weather and this increases the probability of injury as well as stress.

Fencing for weanlings is critical. It should be at least five feet high. Never pasture weanlings in barb wire fencing. There are any number of fencing materials available and you can choose whatever suits your needs as long as it is safe for weanlings. Weanlings love to run and play and many times will run into a fence and this is the reason why it needs to be not only secure, but safe. (The same reasoning applies to sucklings as to why they should never be around electric fencing.) If the donkeys shelter is a run-in shed, it needs to be well bedded to encourage the weanlings to sleep inside, especially in inclement weather. Wood shavings are a preferred bedding material.

Weanlings should have been vaccinated at 3 months or 4 months of age. One vaccination called a 5 in 1 consists of A1 and A2 Influenza, Tetanus and E/W Encephalomyelitis. Respiratory diseases are a problem with weanlings and it is extremely important to vaccinate for Rhinopneumonitis, commonly called Rhino. This vaccination alone can and will save you many veterinarian bills. Weanlings and yearlings routinely have what is commonly known as "the snots" and vaccinating for Rhino will help prevent these problems from getting serious.

> **The Equine Comfort Zone**
>
> **"Should we put the donkeys in tonight?" Usually *you* ask this question when you feel cold. I see my donkeys most comfortable and playful when it's 35 to 40 degrees. So when you are grabbing your coat, your donkey may just be getting comfortable.**
> **In the wild, donkeys would seek out natural shelter such as trees and hillsides. Leaving your barn open at all times, leaves your donkeys the option of going inside when they feel the need.**

Weanlings should also be on a regular deworming program every 30 to 60 days. A paste wormer is easy to administer to weanlings and results in little stress.

Nutrition is also significant during the winter. The growth rate of weanlings is slower than sucklings, but it is still high. This growth rate requires considerable energy, protein, minerals and vitamins. A mixture of one half alfalfa and one half grass hay for weanlings is recommended. (This hay may be too rich and too fattening for adult donkeys, however, is a good hay to feed to donkeys who need weight gain.) During wet weather, hay should be fed inside. Always keep a salt block in front of donkeys.

Keep an eye on hooves. Long hooves on weanlings not only cause crooked legs, but are prone to seedy toe and abscesses. Long hooves can also be like sleds on icy ground and are dangerous to young animals who love to run and play. Many breeders also spread sand around automatic outside waterers and other walkways to keep ice to a minimum and provide good footing.

When You Get Your New Foal Home

We give a halter with the sale of every donkey. NEVER leave a halter on any age donkey when you put them out to pasture. There have been numerous reports of people finding their donkeys laying in the pasture with their back leg entangled in the halter when they went to scratch and got hung up.

We suggest that you spend as much time as you can with your weanling the first several days. Our donkeys are very people and animal oriented and will become very depressed, and possibly ill, if they are totally ignored and kept alone. Your donkey may be a little stand-offish for the first few days until they get to know you. You should pet and rub them as much as possible for the first few days. Donkeys love to have their lower chest scratched.

FEED - Your weanling should b fed two cups of grain (sweet feed) in the evenings. He should be fed this for his first year. After that, if he is in good weight, you can stop the sweet feed or only give them a limited amount as a treat. We feed our weanlings a horse sweet feed)12-13% protein) that can be purchased in any feed store. Our donkeys are fed a hay that contains a mixture of alfalfa and grass. Alfalfa is delicious to donkeys so if your hay does not contain it, they may not each much of it for the first few days until they realize that is all they are going to get. Weanling donkeys can eat as much hay as they want without getting fat.

WATER - Donkeys will not drink stale or dirty water. They must have fresh water daily.

TRAINING - If you want to teach your new donkey to lead, wait at least two weeks before doing so. Let them become accustomed to you and their new home first. Foals have a very short attention span. Your training sessions should never last more than 15 minutes at a time. Foals like to play with people the same way they play with other foals - nipping. If your foal nips you, very quickly pinch his nose. You want to show him that biting you - hurts him. Do not slap your donkey in the face as it will make him very head shy and they usually never get over this. It is important that you do not let jack foals get away with nipping. This behavior should be corrected as soon as it starts.

CASTRATION - You may have your jack foal castrated at any time. We suggest that you wait for a few months. Many people buy their first donkey from us and it is a jack foal. It normally doesn't take long for them to fall in love and want to get into the donkey breeding business! If you do decide to castrate, make an appointment with your vet to have him examine your jack to make sure that both testicles are down. If they are not, your vet cannot castrate him. Some jacks do not mature in this way until they are a year old.

Training Foals

If you have a secure place to work with your jennet and foal, it will make training easier. A large open pasture is just about the worse. The first thing to keep in mind when handling a young donkey is that you will have to deal with their child-like behavior. They can be very playful and will probably try to treat you like a donkey playmate by kicking and biting or rearing at you. Until you are able to catch, halter and control the foal, you just have to try to avoid its antics and discipline it with a loud "NO!". Do not use physical violence on a foal. If the foal rears at you, give it an unbalancing push on the shoulder, making it stagger but not fall, meanwhile saying "NO!" again. Just do NOT make the mistake of encouraging any of this "cute" behavior. Watch the dam and foal - she disciplines him when he bothers her too much. She usually will bite him across the tops of his front legs. This is a good place for a small switch to be used on youngstock as it mimics the mother's discipline practices.

To begin training the foal, you need a physical and mental relationship. If you are able to lift the foal and carry it around at first this will be a big help. It knows then that you can control it and even lift it off its feet but will not hurt it. Try to get it to allow you to pet every part of its body, including between its legs, under its tail, belly and legs. Find its favorite "itch spots" and scratch them. Two favorites are the top of the rump just where the tail joins on and the chest. When the foal is a month or two old, fit a small, well fitting halter with a long soft rope onto the foal. You should lift the foals feet every day from day one. At first the halter will scare him so restrain him with your hands also. Be careful to not lift the feet too high or throw him off balance and scare him.

Once the foal will stand still to be petted and handled all over, you can begin to teach him to lead. Remember, he doesn't know what you want. See if you can get him to take a few steps - perhaps following him mom. Stop, and scratch his favorite spot. Have your beginning lessons inside a small enclosure - the sight of freedom may make him try to run and start a fight that is not good for either of you.

Have a helper lead his mother a few steps at a time and you follow her with the foal. The first few days, when he fights, stop his mother and him and soothe him by talking, scratching and perhaps letting him nurse. The idea is to be persistent but not tire him by more than a few minutes twice a day with these lessons. Small foals are only babies and they tire easily.

NEVER LEAD BY GETTING AHEAD AND PULLING. Stand by the side of the neck and lead the way. Never stop a lesson on a bad note if you can possibly help it. Have the donkey do something right even if it was not what you were trying to teach him before you put him away.

Biting Foals and Adults

There are two major types of biters. The first is a young donkey (most common with intact jacks) that uses the nipping to release pent-up energy. This donkey is often fun and playful but tends to get very impatient. It is important to be firm with this young donkey and to "nip the problem in the bud," but you do not need to reprimand this donkey harshly. This form of nipping is actually "come on, let's play!" rather than "I am going to get you."

The second type of donkey is usually more mature and has a history of being abused. He has turned to biting as a protective mechanism and cannot yet differentiate between friend and foe. He feels that all humans are out to hurt him, and he will try to get you before you can get him. This behavior cannot be permitted, yet it can be difficult to rid this donkey of the vice completely. Regardless, you should be patient and committed to bring about the maximum amount of reform possible.

Occasionally you will find a third type of biter. This donkey nipped as a youngster, and the previous trainer or handler smacked the donkey on the nose as a method of training. This donkey has turned biting into a game. He tries to get you as fast as possible, then sees how many ways he can find to avoid punishment. While not being mean, this type of biter can still be destructive. He will also tend to be head shy because of the hit-and-miss game that he has played in the past. Handling about the head and muzzle can be helpful in curbing this evasive response, but be careful that you are not bitten in the process.

Biting is fairly common among donkeys in the wild. Most donkeys can be broken of the habit, but others will be biters for life. The best solution is to prevent and catch the problem at a very early age. The motivation behind the biting and the current age of the donkey determine how much reform can occur. Even if you cannot completely break your donkey of this habit, you can take steps to reduce the problem. This will at least minimize the chance of injury to yourself or someone else.

When it comes to training your donkey not to bite, there are as many tricks of the trade as there are donkeys that bite. When working with your biter, you do not turn your back on him when you are within his reach, and never let him "play" with your zipper or the sleeve of your coat. More often than not, this is an entre' to a nip. Also be careful when you are grooming any donkey that is known to bite. He may be waiting for you to turn your back and may get you where you least expect it. When you are leading a donkey that bites, pay attention to where you place your lead hand. Many biters will try to eat your hand as they walk. The biter has perfected the art of biting and then pulling away, and he is lightning fast. Keep your eyes open around this donkey or you may end up with less skin than you started with.

When you are training your biter, never hit him on the nose. This will inevitably lead to the head-shy problem described earlier. Smack him on the shoulder, on the rump, under the stomach, but not on the nose. *(Ed Note: You often see jennets correcting their very young foals by nipping them on the front legs in the forearm area. Considering that they are already used to being corrected in this area, you may also use this portion of the body to smack.)* It will solve nothing and will turn into a battle of the quickest. The best approach is to catch your donkey when he is thinking about it but has yet to strike. A sharp "no" or "quit" should make him think otherwise. If he does manage to get in a strike, slap him with the flat of your hand on the neck or shoulder (or on any large body part within reach). Repeat the command "no". Your donkey needs to know that you mean it when you warn him. You must be firm and consistent with this donkey. There is not room for "I'll let you get away with that one but don't do it again." Be vigilant and reprimand at each and every attempted bite. This especially holds true for the more mature donkey that has biting ingrained into his every thought. No matter where he is or who is handling him, do not allow him to bite or even attempt to bite.

Hand feeding your biter is also a no-no. Biting behavior can be exacerbated or even caused by hand feeding treats. We all know that a donkey is never satisfied by one treat alone, and his greed will usually lead to a certain amount of grabbiness. The more grabby he gets, the more he will reach for the hand. Out of frustration, he will grab at any hand, hoping that a treat is enveloped in it. If this happens enough, a biter is created. This is not to say that you have to withhold treats. Just be sure to place any and all treats for a biter in the donkey's feeder rather than feeding him by hand.

Handle your biter as much as possible around his nose and head. Be cautious, but rub his nose, chin, and jowl and let him know that handling can be a pleasurable experience. This will build trust with your donkey and will let him know that he doesn't have to be so self-protective around you.

In regards to biting jacks, much of it is instinctual. Jacks are born with strong herding and protective instincts. It was up to the jack to protect the members of his herd and to defend against intruders. Biting was an indispensable weapon in his arsenal.

Ed Note: Another training device that many donkey owners have used is holding a sharp object in your hand and letting the donkey *run into* it with his mouth as he goes to bite you. Do not jab at the donkey, as the idea is to let the donkey run into the object so that he gets the idea that attempting to bite *you* hurts *him*. The object should not be pointed enough where it would cut or puncture the donkey's skin and it should not be anything that has rust on it.

Reference: Horse Training Basics

Chapter 9

Jacks

A Little About Jacks

There are breeders with very mild mannered jacks who do have success running them with jennets and foals, etc. as a family group. However, I would venture to say these are in the minority and they certainly run a great risk depending on the jack never to change his behavior and become aggressive.

In 21 years as a breeder, I have never run jacks with my jennets all the time. There are many reasons for my decision to segregate the sexes at Windy Ridge Farm, but the main ones are:

Many pasture bred jacks can be very rough on the jennets. Even when in standing heat such jack will often chase and bite jennets unmercifully. Maiden, new or visiting jennets can be quite terrorized and consequently driven to run into fences or jump them, in an effort to escape.

Mature jacks can become very aggressive and harass jennets almost continually whether they are bred or not. Such constant bullying and sometimes attempts at further breeding, can cause abortions to occur.

This same harassing behavior may also be seen if a jennet is left to foal in the same pasture as the jack (NEVER!). With the hormonal changes during the birth process, combined with other smells at foaling time, it is possible a jack may confuse the process with that of a jennet coming in season.

If left with the herd when the jennets are due to foal, some jacks will look upon the arrival of the foal, <u>especially a jack foal,</u> as an intruder. Not only will he then try to get at the foal, but he may kill it if he does reach it.

If left with the herd when jennets foal, then the jack will likely rebreed the jennets when they come into foal heat (7-10 days after foaling). Equine research has shown that such early rebreeding is followed by a high abortion rate - the jennet's reproductive tract is simply not healed sufficiently to sustain another conception. It is preferable to wait for rebreeding until the second or third heat after foaling depending on the condition of mother and foal.

I have always preferred to keep my jennets, foals and youngstock entirely separate from my jacks. Pasture breeding may be the least labor intensive method, but involves the greatest risk, and I have always considered my donkeys to be too important to put them at such risk. Consequently our breeding is always in-hand breeding or equine AI. Either way we have accurate, exact dates on which to predict foaling the following year. That does not however, mean that we isolate our jacks and treat them like lepers! Far from it, because such isolation only promotes the development of abnormal stallion behaviors.

In winter our jacks are kept in alternate large board fence corrals topped with hot wire. Each corral has a run-in box stall in the barn. The alternate corrals between the jacks are home to weanling jacks or jennets who are segregated by sex at the time of weaning (4 - 5 months). At no time are mature breeding jacks ever kept in corrals side by side!

In spring I always have one open jennet destined as companion for each jack, aside from the others he will breed. He will be allowed to hand breed her every second day then, as she is going out of heat, the pair will be put out in their pasture for the summer. I try very hard to chose a jennet that I know he likes and will not boss the jack around - some jennets can be VERY bossy. Some jacks have very definite preferences as to who they will or will not associate with! Our pastures are so arranged that there are at least one or two empty paddocks between one jack and the next.

Reference: Written by Sybil Sewell

Ed Note: For new owners, the breeding process between a jack and jennet can be quite shocking. You raised your sweet little boy from a foal and just know he wouldn't hurt a flea and are totally astonished as to what he can turn into when put in with a jennet in heat - or even jennets who are not in heat. Unfortunately, jacks have this thing about conquering their jennets. That means a lot of chasing and biting. My advice is to never ever put a jack in with a jennet the first time without a muzzle. The breeding process in donkeys is something you'll have to get used to.

MDT Exclusive: Cryptorchidism

So you want to know the truth...

There's been a lot of talk about cryptorchidism (retained testicle) within the Miniature Donkey industry lately. Speculations, rumors and incorrect information has been distributed so ***MDT*** wanted to get the most up-to-date and correct information straight from the *horse's* mouth. With the help of my equine surgeon, I interviewed Dr. John Hurtgen, DVM, ***President*** of the American College of Theriogenology (the study of animal reproductive diseases).

MDT Editor: Please tell me something about cryptorchidism.

Dr. Hurtgen: Cryptorchidism is an hereditary trait. The problem comes in that, and I can't tell you off hand, what the mode of inheritance is, but its not a straight forward dominant type of inheritance. In other words, it's not so much that the stallion is a cryptorchid he needs to carry the gene for cryptorchidism. He may or may not in fact be a cryptorchid and the mother of the resulting foal also has to have some combination of genes also and then you will produce a high incidence of cryptorchidism. There's one farm in Texas that has two stallions that they stand at stud. One is a cryptorchid and one is not. About half of the colts out of the normal stallion are cryptorchid and about a fourth of the colts out of the cryptorchid stallion turn out to be cryptorchid. Both of his stallions carry the gene for cryptorchidism and both of his stallions are abnormal. Again, cryptorchidism is hereditary but many cryptorchid stallions that are at stud are bred to mares that don't have that gene in their background, may never produce resulting foals, but if the resulting offspring then somewhere down the line are then bred to a horse with the cryptorchid gene then you are likely to see a slew of them.

MDT Editor: If you breed a cryptorchid jack, mainly because you are trying to reproduce a certain color, to his daughters, is the cryptorchid gene then doubled?

Dr. Hurtgen: Yes, a lot of their male offspring will be cryptorchid.

MDT Editor: If a son out of a cryptorchid jack has both testicles, what are the chances of his producing cryptorchid sons of his own? Then again, I suppose it would depend on if the jennet carried the cryptorchid gene wouldn't it.

Dr. Hurtgen: Yes, that's correct. Just because the sire is cryptorchid doesn't mean he will pass the cryptorchidism condition to his son. Let me see if I can give you an example. Say you have a male red rose and a female white rose and you breed them four times. You will end up with one red rose, two pink roses and one white rose.

Cryptorchid Male		Female
Red Rose	***BRED TO:***	White Rose
RR		rr

Produces
Rr (Pink)

Breed Two Pink Roses (Rr, Rr)-Four Times:

	Produces		
RR	rr	Rr	rR
Red	White	Pink	Pink

If the jack you want to breed to happens to have the genes of the white rose (rr) and another white rose (rr) even though it resulted from two pink breedings, you would have no chance of producing a Red (RR) rose. IF the colt you want to breed to happens to have the genes of Rr so to speak and you mated them to another Rr maybe you would end up one fourth of the time having a normal colt with two testicles, half the time you'd have a colt with two testicles but he'd carry the genetic factor for cryptorchidism, so when you subsequently bred that jack that has two testicles but really he's carrying gene for cryptorchidism, half of his resulting offspring would be carriers, one fourth would actually be cryptorchid and one fourth would be okay and not have the gene. That's a lot.

The genetics for cryptorchidism isn't quite that simple. It's two or three gene combinations that produce cryptorchidism.

MDT Editor: How do you feel about people using cryptorchid stallions as sires?
Dr. Hurtgen: Well, I don't know about the miniature donkey industry but you see the horse industry is not driven by economics. It's driven by non-economic factors therefore it is very difficult for a breed association to do anything about somebody who wants to stand a horse that carries a genetic defect, other than education. Of course the genes get spread within the gene pool. In the Quarter Horse for example there are certain sire lines that are pretty popular in which we see a fair number of cryptorchid foals every year and we see a lot of umbilical hernias in certain sire lines so umbilical hernias are also hereditary. Parrot mouth and offset knees are also hereditary.

MDT Editor: This is the problem with miniature donkeys because my guess is that there are under 10,000 miniature donkeys in the U.S. and Canada. I know of one jack who has produced quite a number of cryptorchid sons that people purchased as babies and didn't know that the weanling was carrying this defect.

Dr. Hurtgen: Well, these people didn't have to buy them, they could have had the jack examined.

MDT Editor: Well, how would they know if they purchased them as weanlings?

Dr. Hurtgen: Well, a normal colt has two testicles at birth. Now there are times when a colt is born with only one testicle but by the time he's six months old the second testicle will descend. I have had a few horses as old as 4 years old drop the second testicle even though he had just one up until that time. In a horse that drops that second testicle at the age of 2, 3, 4 years of age that horse may be carrying exactly the same gene as the horse with one testicle and always has one testicle. However, the normal situation, is for a foal at birth - at one day of age - to have two fully descended testicles. That's what is considered normal. There are supposedly horses that have two descended testicles, let's say until they are six months or a year old then all of a sudden a two years old, boom, they're gone. Now, the documentation of that is kind of difficult to come by. When a horse turns out to be a cryptorchid as a two year old and then you go back to the guy who owned the horse when he was a foal and say "hey, do you remember if this horse had two testicles when he was a baby?" Oh sure, he had two testicles. Well, see the horse may or may not have been specifically checked for two normal testicles in his scrotum.

It's a shame to have these genes continue to be bred into the miniature donkeys since you have such a small gene pool to begin with. In mammoth jacks there has been the importation of semen from Spain, Poland, etc into the United States to introduce totally different genetics but apparently you don't have that option.

Castration

This is the name given to the surgery which changes a stallion into a gelding and renders him unreproductive by removal of the testicles. The procedure is also referred to as "gelding".

Donkey and horses are castrated for several reasons. Removing the testicles eliminates the source of male hormones in the body. This takes away the animal's sex drive, resulting in an animal who acts more like a mare than like a stallion. This allows the gelding, as the resulting animal is called, to be used around jennets/mares without undesirable breeding behavior. It also makes the animal much safer to handle and to be around.

A gelding usually has a more consistent disposition. Another very

important reason for castration is to keep inferior animals from reproducing; this is important to the improvement of all breeds of animals, not just horses. As with many other types of surgery, the earlier it is done, the easier it is on the animal. Donkeys and horses may be castrated at a few weeks of age. There is a problem with this procedure at such an early age. The resulting gelding often has thin poorly developed front quarters, neck, and head. For this reason, most people wait until the animal is at least a year of age.
The difference between doing the surgery at one year and at two years of age is somewhat a matter of personal preference. Veterinarians often get a batch of stud colts to castrate in the spring of their two-year old year. As the animals begin to come to sexual maturity, they try to cross fences to get to jennets and mares that they can smell, often severely injuring themselves in the process. At this point, the owner will often suddenly decide that he doesn't have the facilities to keep the animal, or does not want the animal for breeding purposes.

Many ranchers castrate their own horse colts. This is generally a rough-and-ready rodeo, with the animals roped and tied down and some cowboy wielding a sharp knife. My opinion is that this is a rather barbaric way to do a major operation on an animal as sensitive as a horse. For that reason, this article does not include a description or how to castrate your own animal. It is worth the price to most owners to have the surgery done under anesthesia to lessen the animal's suffering. A final word on this point - the shock resulting from the excitement combined with the pain of the surgery can kill a horse. That makes a veterinary bill look small in comparison.

THE OPERATION

The animal should be in good health when the surgery is done. He should not be recently recovered from any serious disease, especially distemper. Be sure to tell your veterinarian if the animal has been on sweet clover pasture or has been fed sweet clover hay, as these feeds may make the animal more prone to bleeding. The animal should not have been recently wormed, especially not with organophosphate wormers; some of these make the animal more susceptible to some of the anesthetics that are used and may cause serious complications. If at all possible, surgery should be done in spring or fall, either before fly season, or after a frost has killed most of the flies. Most veterinarians do not like to castrate donkey and horses during cold, rainy weather. Not only is it miserable work, but it seems to me that animals have more complications if castrated during these periods.

Veterinarians give some sort of anesthetic before starting to castrate. Your veterinarian has developed a routine which works for him. This may range from a small dose of tranquilizer and local anesthetic injected directly into the spermatic cords and nerves as he does surgery with the animal standing, to completely anesthetizing the donkey or horse until he is flat on the ground. He may or may not tie the animal up after it is asleep. He will then make incision - usually one over each testicle - and remove the testicles. He uses a clamp called an emasculator to crush the cords and blood vessels. This helps to prevent bleeding from the surgery site. After the testicles are removed, many veterinarians open the scrotal sack as far as they possibly can. This is to allow the area to drain well and to help prevent swelling and complications.

(Ed Note: It has previously been reported to MDT that miniature donkeys have had a problem with excessive bleeding. The castration instrument, called an emasculator, has both a "crimper" and a "cutter". The crimper is ready-made for the large spermatic cord of the horse stallion. The spermatic cord of the miniature donkey, while not anatomically different, is smaller than the stallion. In some cases the crimper may not properly compress the cord, causing it to bleed when cut. The vet MUST be sure the cord is properly compressed, taking into account it's smaller size. DO NOT assume your vet is aware of this, so bring it to his attention.)

COMPLICATIONS AFTER CASTRATION

BLEEDING

Bleeding often occurs from the edges of the cut on the scrotum; it may also occur from a small artery in the spermatic cord. The donkey or horse may appear to bleed quite heavily, especially in warm weather. Untying the animal, if he has been restrained, and allowing him to relax will help reduce his blood pressure (which has been raised by the excitement and handling). This in itself helps the bleeding to stop. It rarely lasts more than 5 minutes. A small amount of dripping (a drop to a few drops at a time) beyond this time is not a problem. If the animal appears to be bleeding heavily more than an hour after surgery, consult your veterinarian and have him recheck the animal to make sure there are no problems or complications.

SWELLING

Swelling of the scrotal area may occur after castration, as well as swelling of the animal's penis, sheath, and hind legs. The animal may be reluctant to move; when forced to do so, he may move stiffly with a straddling gait. He may have an elevated temperature and little or no appetite. These complications can be almost entirely prevented by adequate exercise after castration to help keep the circulation moving in the area and to remove infected material.

If severe swelling occurs, call your veterinarian AT ONCE so that he may reopen the area, clean it out, and get it to draining adequately. He may wish to put the animal on antibiotics for a period of time. If he does use antibiotics, be sure to give the prescribed amount of medication for the correct length of time. Failure to dose may lengthen the animal's recovery time or result in his dying from infection. This problem can largely be prevented by adequate exercise after the surgery. If you have an animal swollen like this, it is probably your own fault. By trying to be "kind" to him, you have caused him a considerable amount of extra pain and discomfort and possibly endangered his life.

AFTERCARE

Some veterinarians administer penicillin after surgery; others do not. This is a matter of personal preference; a single dose probably does more for the owner's peace of mind than it does for the possibility of infection. If your donkey has not had a recent booster of tetanus toxoid, the veterinarian may administer either this or tetanus antitoxin, depending on the donkey's immunization history. If it is fly season, it will be necessary to spray the surgical area daily with a good fly spray. Don't spray it directly into the wound unless the flies are so bad that this is absolutely necessary. For most animals, spraying the vicinity is good enough.

Aftercare by the owner does more to prevent swelling and infection than anything the veterinarian can do. It is of the utmost importance to give the animal adequate exercise after surgery. This helps the opened area to rub together and drain out blood clots, as well as helping to remove infected material if there is any. It prevents swelling. If left to himself, the new gelding may stay in one place, nursing his sore spots. The worst possible thing that you as an owner can do is to just allow the horse to stand and become swollen. If a significant amount of swelling occurs, your veterinarian may have to re-anesthetize the animal and reopen and clean the wound. Some donkeys who have been allowed to stand will swell up to an enormous size. Needless to say, they will be in misery. The local swelling is usually accompanied by edema of the hind legs, often called "stocking" or "stocking up."

How much exercise should you give the animal? My personal policy is to let the animal rest on the day he is castrated. The day after, the owner is to exercise him 30 minutes to an hour. The second day after surgery, an hour is the absolute MINIMUM! Two hours are even better, continuing this amount of work DAILY until the animal is completely healed, which usually takes about two weeks. What kind of work? Spend that time walking him. Spending some of the time at a trot or a lope is even better.

Do NOT assume that since your donkey has been castrated, it is safe to turn him in with jennet and mares who are in heat. While sperm cells are no longer produced by the testicles, live semen may remain in some of the glands of the reproductive system for several weeks. Thus, the donkey or horse may be fertile enough to get a jennet or mare pregnant - usually the one you DIDN'T want bred. Assume an absolute MINIMUM of ten days for all fertile sperm to die. Two to three weeks are even better if you can allow that much time.

Also, it takes a period of time for the hormones to leave the animal's body. He may exhibit stallion-like behavior for a varying period of time, depending on how rapidly these are removed from the bloodstream. This usually requires a few days to a few weeks, depending on the individual. It also depends on how old the animal was when castrated. An older stallion may retain sexual behavior for a longer period of time than a younger animal would who was not fixed in this behavior pattern.

Reference: Written by Ruth B. James, DVM

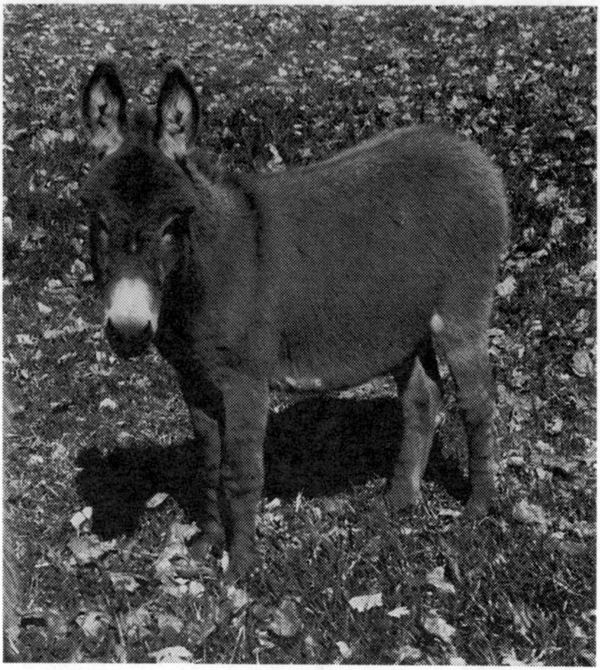

Chapter 10

Miscellaneous Health Care

Laboratory Tests for Donkeys

"I don't want to spend any more money than is necessary," my client grumbled. "Why should I have a blood test done on my donkey? It's obvious that he just has a cold." Why, indeed? Many donkeys suffer brief bouts of the flu or mild cases of colic, recovering quickly without further incident. Your vet comes out, administers some type of medication, and that's all there is to the matter. Or is it?

What about that case of the flu that turns into pneumonia? Or the case of colic that recurs frequently and mysteriously? At what point should the veterinarian look beyond the physical exam and ask for further testing?

The myth of the veterinarian who can diagnose with one quick glance continues to persist, despite all the advantages of modern medicine and new technology. Old Dr. Ben, he was a good one. Knew exactly the problem with a quick physical exam, and supplied the treatment just as quickly.

In the old days, there wasn't much in the way of treatment choices, nor was there much knowledge about specific diseases. But our diagnostic abilities have grown by leaps and bounds. We now know more about different disease processes, and have a huge arsenal of treatment regimens to choose from. Yet the choice of an optimal treatment depends on exactly what the problem happens to be.

When should laboratory tests be done? The most obvious time is when your donkey is suffering from a severe illness. Another indication for testing is when a medical problem occurs over time or more than once—the donkey which colics frequently, has muscle soreness after light exercise, or is losing weight for no apparent reason.

When and how often tests are done also depends on you, the donkey owner. Are you comfortable with your veterinarian's "almost 95% sure" diagnosis, or would you prefer documented proof? Would you rather use the medication which most often works on the majority of donkeys with a respiratory infection, or do you want to know what medicine will work for sure?

If you elect to go for a test, the results may simply confirm that the treatment indicated is that which your vet recommended. If your donkey is the exception to the rule, though, you'll be ahead in time and money because you'll know that the routine medication wouldn't have worked, and your vet will choose a more appropriate medication immediately.

The mainstay of diagnosis continues to be a thorough, accurate physical exam. But we can learn much more about the donkey's body through a wide array of laboratory and blood tests. The exam determines which, if any, of those tests might help the veterinarian select a better treatment for the donkey, or might help narrow down a specific diagnosis of the problem.

THE CBC

The CBC, or complete blood count, is the first laboratory test your veterinarian might call for. In this evaluation, the donkey's blood cells are evaluated and counted. First, the total white blood cell (WBC) count gives an overall picture: is it low, normal, or high?

An increased **white blood cell** count might result from stress, inflammation, or infection. And a decreased count could indicate that the cells are pooling somewhere in the donkey's body.

The **red blood cell** volume is evaluated in relation to the donkey's plasma volume. The relationship between these is expressed as the **hematocrit** or packed cell volume (**PCV**). When the PCV is high, it may indicate that the donkey is dehydrated; if the PCV is low, the donkey may be anemic.

Plasma protein levels are measured next. Protein levels may be high due to chronic inflammation, or low because of diarrhea or other loss.

For the differential white blood cell count, a drop of blood is smeared onto a slide and stained. Here, the different types of white blood cells are closely examined, and their numbers compared to normal. **Neutrophils** are the "pus cells" which come raging to the rescue when your donkey suffers from a bacterial infection. And **lymphocytes** tend to increase in number when a virus invades your donkey's body.

The **eosinophil** is a brightly staining white blood cell which increases in number in response to allergy, irritation, or parasite infestation (worms!). And **monocytes** are found in higher numbers when a disease has been present for a longer period of time.

In the case of respiratory disease, your veterinarian might be searching for several answers: Is the donkey suffering from heaves, an allergic problem? Or does it have a virus, such as influenza? Has the problem existed for some time, gradually creeping up on the donkey so that you only recently noticed? Or is it an acute (sudden) illness?

Comparing blood counts several days apart can help your vet evaluate how well your donkey is combating the disease, and how well the medication is working. A high white blood cell count from pneumonia will begin to drop soon after antibiotics are administered, if that medication was effective against the offending bacteria.

The donkey with colic can also benefit from the CBC. Severe cases of colic will present with a high PCV, due to dehydration or shock, and sometimes will have a very low total WBC count. This is because the white blood cells are pooling in an injured area of the donkey's intestine. And a high number of eosinophils could indicate that the cause of the colic episode was intestinal parasites.

SERUM CHEMISTRIES

Your veterinarian may order a set of blood chemistries from the lab. Your donkey's serum, obtained after the clot is removed from the blood sample, contains many enzymes, proteins, and other substances which are produced by the body's every day functions.

Each of these substances is produced by specific body tissues in particular levels. An increase or decrease in any of the products measured can indicate a problem with a particular part of your donkey's body.

For example, a donkey suffering from muscle soreness might have an increase in the **enzyme creatine kinase (CK).** This enzyme is produced by normal muscle cells; exercise or bruising can cause an increase in blood levels of CK.

Donkeys which suffer from tying up, an abnormal stiffening and soreness of the muscles, will have a greatly elevated CK level. As treatment and a specific training schedule are instituted, the donkey's CK levels are monitored to evaluate how well it's responding.

Many veterinarians will recommend a routine chemistry screen for older donkeys. Some old donkeys lose weight gradually; even though they might need dental work or more groceries, there's often more than that involved. As the donkey ages, its kidney and liver function may start to deteriorate. The chem screen will reflect those problems, and your veterinarian can make specific recommendations on changes in your donkey's diet and overall management.

SEROLOGY

Serology is the study of serum with the purpose of identifying antibodies. Antibodies are specific proteins produced by the donkey to help fight disease. In some cases, serology is the only way to definitively diagnose the donkey's illness.

Potomac donkey fever, influenza, rhinopneumonitis, and equine infectious anemia (EIA) are diseases commonly diagnosed through serology. The test for EIA is familiar to most donkey owners as the Coggins test.

Evidence of antibodies to a specific disease in the donkey's blood is not enough for a diagnosis, however. Those antibodies will be present at some level for a long time. Because of that, two samples are usually taken, several weeks apart. A sharp rise in the antibody level gives a good indication that the infection was, in fact, very recent.

OTHER LABORATORY TESTS

Other fluid and tissue samples can be taken for a detailed look at specific cells, either from a tumor or from body cavities. Donkeys normally have a small amount of fluid in their chest and abdominal cavities, and a sample can be taken to help evaluate illness.

Abdominocentesis is the process of obtaining fluid from the donkey's abdomen, and is commonly done to help evaluate cases of colic. And thoracocentesis involves obtaining chest (thoracic) fluid for evaluation of respiratory disease.

A sample of joint fluid is often taken to check for infection or signs of other joint disease. And a transtracheal wash obtains fluid and cells from the donkey's airway, aiding in the diagnosis of respiratory disease.

The processes used for taking these varied samples are all similar. The area to be evaluated is clipped and surgically scrubbed before a local anesthetic is administered. Next, a needle, biopsy instrument, or catheter is inserted and fluid or cells are aspirated. The amount needed is not large, since even a drop can be placed on a microscope slide and viewed under high power.

First, the type and number of cells are examined. Your veterinarian usually looks at tracheal washes or abdominal fluid immediately. A possible finding might be an increase in **neutrophils** on a tracheal wash, which indicates a bacterial infection.

Other samples are sent to a veterinary pathologist for evaluation. That lump on your donkey's skin must be carefully identified so that the proper treatment can be instituted.

Sometimes cultures are submitted to a laboratory for evaluation of microbial growth. When the type of bacteria causing an infection is known, then the most effective treatment can be chosen.

Cells are not the only substance evaluated in these samples. Levels of protein, glucose (sugar), and other products are measured as well.

Your donkey's urine and manure can provide clues to its health, too. The manure is most often evaluated for numbers and types of parasite eggs. The presence of large amounts of sand in the manure can give a clue to the cause of recurrent colic. Urine samples tell a great deal to the learned observer. First, the urine's concentration, or specific gravity, is measured; this gives clues as to the normal functioning of the donkey's kidneys. Urine can be sent to the lab for bacterial culture if a urinary tract infection is suspected. And the cells present in the donkey's urine can be examined for evidence of disease.

LAB RESULTS

How long should you expect to wait to hear of the results on your donkey's blood or laboratory tests? The answer depends on the test done and upon the location of the laboratory. Samples evaluated by your own veterinarian are often done the same day, while certain laboratories have a one day turn around time. Biopsies, cultures, and some other involved tests may take a week or more. You can expect that any significant findings will be reported immediately to your veterinarian, as soon as they're obtained.

The results of a test may confirm that the proper treatment regimen is being used, or may cause your vet to change some aspect of the donkey's management. Perhaps a different drug will be used, or medications may be administered over a longer time than was originally planned. Sometimes the test results can leave you frustrated. Perhaps the results only confirmed your veterinarian's suspicions, leaving you wondering whether the test was really necessary at all. Or maybe all the test results were normal, and your donkey still has a problem. In both these cases, the tests were still not a waste of time. Often, a set of normal serum chemistries helps to rule out many possible diseases, helping your vet to narrow down the problem. And many times both you and your veterinarian need the reassurance that your treatment regimen is indeed appropriate, and that you just haven't given the donkey enough time to fully recover.

The next time your veterinarian suggests running some laboratory tests on your donkey, give some thought to the matter. What will the tests do to help your donkey? Is further information needed in order to properly treat its illness? Is your donkey's illness severe enough that you need more information quickly? Or is the problem a mild one that gives you the flexibility to wait for tests only if your present treatment doesn't work?

While most of your donkey's medical problems are minor ones, you may need the help of laboratory evaluations one day. And we're certainly fortunate to have such medical expertise available.

Reference: Written by Dr. Carin Smith who has been a practicing veterinarian since 1984.

Dryland Distemper (Pigeon Fever)

Ed Note: We received the following correspondence and photos from one of our readers in California whose donkey came down with Dryland Distemper.

October 10...Today I took some digital photos of Daphne's chest area. I'm sending them by email and hope you are able to "see" the swelling.

Her "breasts" are swollen the size of half-grapefruits. They are quite firm. The area between her front legs is swollen, but soft. Her temperature is 100 degrees. Her appetite for carrots is great. I have given her 1/2g of Bute today. I very gently rub the swollen areas and have applied a heating pad on the low setting twice so far today for 20-minute sessions. I took her and her companion, Jackson, on a 1/2-mile stroll. I felt it would help her spirits and circulation. She did fine, but we were caught in a sudden rainstorm. Of course, they were not happy about being wet. I did bring her in the house, she seemed happy to be there.

October 14 ...Just a quick update on Daphne. Veterinarian Betty Nunes came out yesterday.

She felt it was Pigeon Fever, but asked if we wanted her to do a culture to be certain. We said yes. She withdrew separate samples from the two hardened areas in Daphne's breast.

She sedated Daphne and asked permission to shave the chest areas to be lanced. We agreed. She shaved the two areas and gave Daphne a local anesthetic. She made two deep 1 1/2" incisions in the swollen areas. She had my daughter hold a bag underneath the incisions while she "expressed" a mixture of pus and blood from each area. My husband estimated that approximately 4 oz of material came from each area. The vet did not want to get this on the ground as it would be a contaminant. We need to flush out the wounds with a saline/mild povidone solution twice a day. She advises 1/2g bute twice a day. We will hear back on the culture by the end of the week.

She advises fly spray for all of our horses & donkeys (we usually do this anyway) and SWAT around the perimeter of any wounds or scabs. Unfortunately, we had to remove Daphne's companion donkey, Jackson, from the area until she recovers. The vet was worried that he might get it. Daphne is doing well this morning. She really loves to put her head in your arms and be rubbed.

October 16 ...Daphne is doing well, although the incisions look pretty gruesome. Yes, there has been continuing drainage from the incisions. My husband flushes them out twice daily and I keep SWAT around the perimeter. I am thinking of modifying a large fly mask to protect the chest area. The culture came back, it is definitely Pigeon Fever. The vet felt that the bacteria could continue to live in the soil if we allowed the infected drainage material to drop onto the ground. Also flies could transmit the infected material to other equines.

The vet is coming back on Friday to check her. She felt the prognosis was good although it could take 10-12 days for this to run its course. The wounds need to heal from the inside out.

Daphne is braying again; she tries to kick me when I attempt to take her temperature; she will only take the BUTE if it is hidden in whole wheat bread; her appetite is good. We are encouraged, but it is very difficult to see her go through this.

Dryland Distemper (Pigeon Fever)

Horses in arid regions of the Western states are most at risk for this disease. We can blame this disease on a very talented bacteria called "Corynebacterium pseudotuberculosis", which can cause a lot of problems in different animals. Dryland distemper is also known as pigeon fever due to the development of abscesses in the ventral and pectoral region. The chest and underbelly become swollen, then abscesses form in these areas within one to four weeks. Other clinical signs include anorexia, lethargy, fever, lameness. The duration of the disease varies from weeks to months, depending on the severity of the abscesses.

Most abscesses occur under the skin of the chest or along the underbelly, but can also form in the arm pits and sheath, near mammary glands and on the legs. The bacteria is also capable of entering the bloodstream and forming internal abscesses inside the chest and abdomen. If these internal abscesses rupture, it is usually fatal. Luckily, this rarely happens. While reoccurrence is possible, most horses get the disease only once.

The bacteria that causes dryland distemper also causes "caseous lymphagitis" in sheep and goats and "ulcerative lymphagitis" in cattle and horses. It has also been found in deer and in the ticks that feed on deer. For these reasons, dryland distemper has appeared in areas where infected sheep and goats are present. It is uncertain how contagious it is or how it is transmitted, but biting flies and insects are suspected.

Dryland distemper occurs in arid regions of the western United States, with California having a high percentage of the cases. The disease can occur anytime during the year, but most cases occur during the fall and early winter months. At this time, there are no effective vaccines to prevent this disease, and only moderately effective antibiotics to treat it once the animal contracts the disease.

Daphne 10/10/97

7 year old miniature donkey

9 hands tall

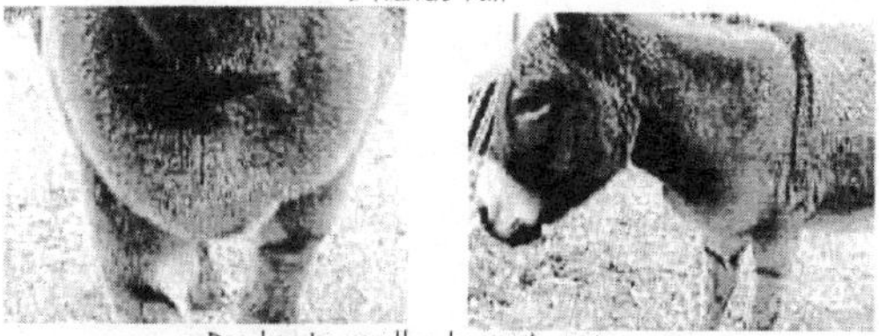

Daphne's swollen breast area

10/10/97

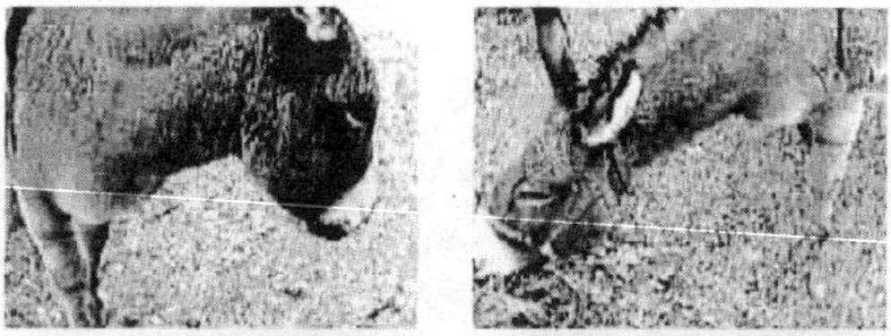

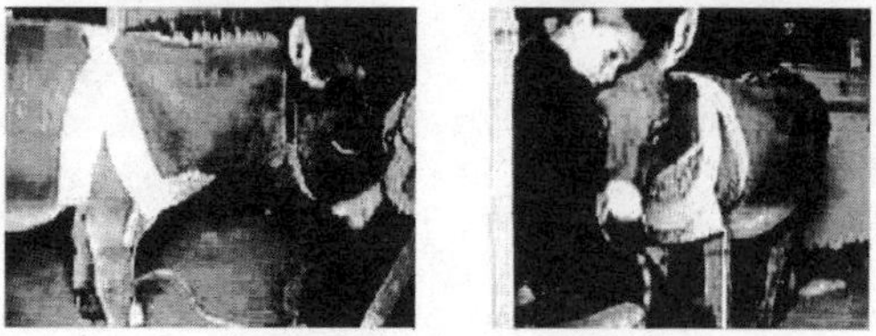

heating pad on low setting held

with large ACE bandage

Upward Fixation of the Patella

"Patella" is the technical name for the kneecap. In the normal equine, it rides in a groove in the lower end of the femur exactly like your kneecap or mine. An affected equine has the kneecap slide upward and "catch", causing his leg to lock straight rather than being able to bend normally. The problem can be hereditary in animals with overly straight, upright hind legs. Fixation can also occur because the animal is injured while the leg was overextended. *Animals who* are *weakened and thin are more prone* to *it than are animals in normal condition.* Fixation generally is seen in only one hind leg at a time, but often occurs in either hind leg in susceptible animals. It is common in Shetland ponies and has been seen fairly often in Miniature Donkeys.

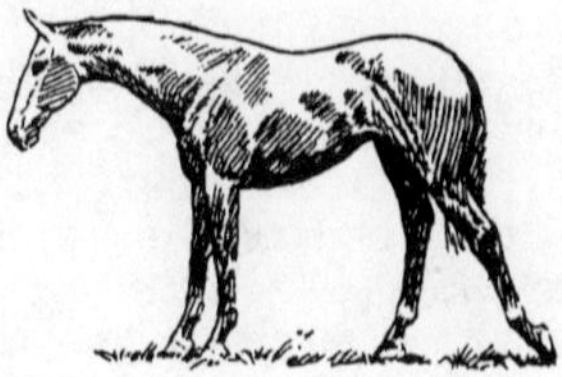

The animal's leg is locked in the extended position, stretched out behind him.

The animal cannot flex the stifle and hock, but can still move the fetlock. The leg may unlock and then catch again in a few steps or it may stay locked for hours or days. Some equine have the kneecap catch as they move, giving a rough, jerky gait, without its ever locking and staying locked. If the animal is forced to move while the patella is locked hard and fast, he may drag the front of the hoof on the ground. A snapping sound can sometimes be heard as the kneecap pops in and out of place without locking.

If fixation happens to your donkey suddenly and does not relieve itself shortly, first-aid to get the kneecap popped back into place may be in order. Pull the leg forward, at the same time, push the kneecap toward the donkey's body. This will often push it back into place. Other animals benefit by being backed while someone pushes inward and downward on the kneecap. In mild cases of fixation of the patella, where a donkey only occasionally locks up, the donkey appears uncomfortable. In severe cases, where an operation is needed, the donkey shows mild pain and is somewhat reluctant to run and play and has an overall appearance of being depressed.

Special Editors Note: I purchased a jennet foal several years ago (sight unseen) who arrived in poor malnourished condition. Shortly thereafter, both back legs locked up. She was put on a stringent worming program and a high protein/vitamin feed program. We also did daily physical therapy on her back legs. We were advised that with proper exercise and nutrition, there was a possibility for her to outgrow this condition. She improved greatly, however, as a yearling both her back legs continued to lock so we opted for surgery. The surgical correction for upward fixation of the patella is a "medial patellar desmotomy."

Medial Patellar Desmotomy
The surgical site is shaved and scrubbed with an antiseptic, and a local anesthetic is injected into the area. The jennet was tranquilized and in a standing position. A small incision was made over the middle patellar ligament, through which a knife is placed underneath the medial patellar ligament. The knife blade is turned so that its sharp edge is against the ligament which is then severed. One suture was used to close the small incision in each leg.

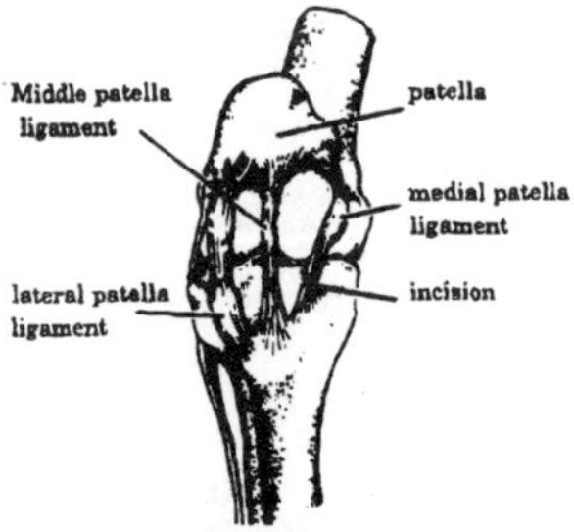

Medial Patellar Desmotomy

Important Note: The medial patellar ligament will eventually grow back together over a three month period of time. I spoke with several other breeders who had this procedure done, and in most cases, the operation was not a success. All other breeders advised that they were told to stall their donkeys for several weeks and eliminate as much exercise as possible. My equine surgeon, on the other hand, advised me the exact opposite. He wanted me to begin

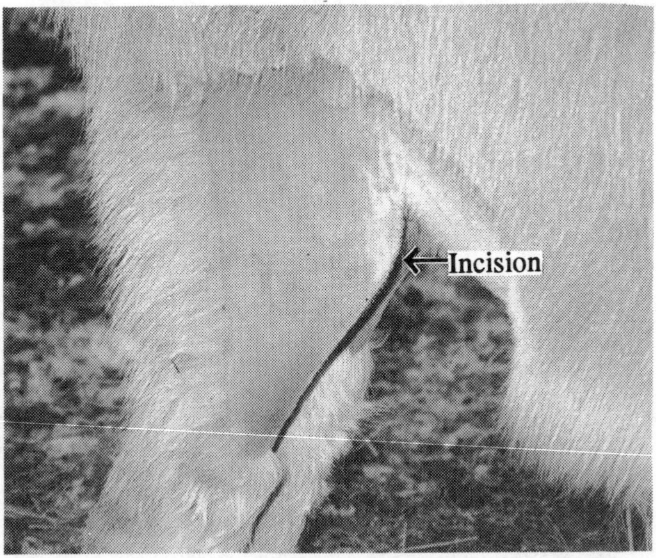

exercise the very next day - preferably by trotting the jennet up hills. The purpose of this was to build up the hind leg muscles. These muscles would help hold the patellar ligament in place as it grew back together. This jennet was given the proper exercise and I deemed the operation an 80% success. I say 80% because this jennet did occasionally lock up to the point where she jerks the hind leg up. She does not totally lock and I saw no evidence of pain. Now four years later it's a very rare occasion to see her lock up at all. I firmly believe the fact that we exercised this animal had a great deal to do with the success of this particular operation. I also feel this condition had caused this jennet a good amount of stress. She was always very laid back, however after the operation, turned into a very playful and much happier animal. I might also mention that I have seen jennets in their last month of pregnancy occasionally lock up and feel there must be a correlation between the extra added weight and stress that is put on the ligaments during this time frame. The fees for this procedure were: $10 -Tranquilizer, $150 - Surgery, $10 - Two sutures, and $5 - Tetanus Toxoid for a total cost of $175.00.

Anemia

Anemia is not a disease in and of itself, and there are very few signs associated with anemia unless it is severe. It's usually a component of another disease process.

There are some unique features of equine physiology that complicate the accurate diagnosis of anemia. The most important, is the splenic reserve of red blood cells. Horses at rest store as much as 30% of their RBC's in the spleen, a large muscular organ on the left side of the abdomen. When the animal is exercised or excited, the spleen contracts releasing its reserve of blood cells into the blood stream. At rest the packed cell volume (a commonly made measure for anemia) may be in the low twenties and a diagnosis of anemia made when the animal is perfectly normal. Take the same horse and lunge him aggressively for 5 minutes and his PCV will rise to a normal 35. A horse must be exercised briefly, but aggressively just prior to testing for accurate results.

> **Average red blood cell count on donkeys is 6.1 to 6.3 however can range from 5.0 to 6.9. Normal values for horses is generally 5.5 to 10.5**

The most common cause of anemia in horses is chronic inflammation. In chronic inflammation iron metabolism is altered so that iron released from the normal breakdown of blood cells is not available in the bone marrow production of new blood cells. So you see the hematocrit or the packed cell volume (PCV) drop to the 25-20% range. Normal is 40-45%. That's the percentage of the blood that is red blood cells.

In chronic disease/inflammation cases, the way to treat the anemia is to correct the primary condition - the pneumonia, or pleuritis, or abdominal abscess. As the inflammation subsides, the animal will correct the anemia on its own without any external medications specifically for anemia.

The other causes of anemia are much more uncommon. They include immune-mediated reactions in the adult equine. The mechanism behind that is similar to what is seen in the foals with neonatal erythrolysis, where antibodies are produced against the red blood cells and they are destroyed. That can happen as a side effect of drugs or immune reactions related to infectious diseases, viruses, or bacteria.

Diagnosis

If your donkey/horse is anemic, you will need your vets help in figuring it out as the problem is usually secondary to other troubles. Consider the three main cause of anemia:

1. blood loss
2. hemolysis (RBC rupture)
3. inadequate RBC production.

Both blood loss and hemolysis can either be rapidly developing or chronic disorders and clinical signs will depend on which you have. With mild anemia there may be few signs other than exercise intolerance and poor appearance. Inadequate production tends to be a chronic disorder usually brought on by other diseases. In the acute disorder, weakness, lethargy, and pale mucous membranes develop within a few hours. In the slow developing scenario, the above signs develop over a long time and may be accompanied by weight loss, fever, and poor hair coat.

In blood loss anemia, the anemia is secondary to bleeding which will need to be found and treated. Usually infection or neoplasia are the cause. In the acute bleeding patient, if more than 1 quart of blood per 100 lbs of horse is lost, whole blood transfusions will be necessary.

Nutritional causes of anemia are rare, but starvation may cause it. Unlike humans, iron deficiency anemia is rare in equine. The animals diet is usually rich in iron and iron supplementation for treating anemia is rarely needed and should be avoided, particularly in young foals. Good quality hay or grass is an excellent source of iron.

Infectious causes of anemia include: intestinal parasites, equine infectious anemia (EIA), blood parasites (Babesia), chronic abscesses, staph and clostridia, lice and ticks.

Poisons that may cause anemia are: nitrites, wilted red maple leaves, wild onions, undiluted IV DMSO, chronic lead, arsenic or copper ingestion, and rattlesnake venom.

References: Resources: Portions of this article is provided by The Equineman's Advisor. AAEP - Reprinted portions with permission Fairfield Bain, DVM, MS, Dip. ACVIM, Dip. American College of Pathology, is an internal medicine specialist at Hagyard-Davidson-McGee veterinary firm in Lexington, Ky.

Do Mini Donkeys Get Mini Vaccinations?

Many people ask me if a Miniature Donkey should get a lesser dose of vaccine than the manufacturer recommends for a full-sized horse. Below we quote from a letter written by David Hustead, DVM of Fort Dodge Laboratories when he was asked the same question regarding a miniature horse, and as you know, we vaccinate our mini donkeys the same as horses.

"The immune system of all horses is controlled by its genetic coding. This coding is almost exactly the same in all horses, regardless of size. The immune system in a tiny horse does not know that its body is only the size of a large dog. For all the immune system knows, it could just as easily be in a 1500 pound Shire draft horse.

The currently held theory for vaccine function is that an individual immune system is stimulated by what we call antigenic mass.

The antigenic mass can be compared to the number of BB's in a shot gun shell. If we have enough BB's we can kill our game. If we have enough antigenic mass in a vaccine, then the immune system is stimulated. If not enough antigenic mass is present, then we get no response from the animal in response to our vaccine. Since the immune system in a 350 pound horse is the same immune system that is found in a 1500 pound horse, the both require the same antigenic mass to be stimulated by a vaccine. So, while you are correct that the dose to weight ratio is very high in your miniatures, you can see this is not the important issue as far as we can tell. Until better scientific information is available, I would recommend your miniature get the same dose as vaccine as any other horse."

(Ed Note: Please take notice that this only applies to vaccines such as flu, rhino, tetanus, etc. It does not apply to other drugs such as pain killers, antibiotics, prostaglandin's, etc. These drugs are given by weight. A miniature could easily be killed by giving too much of these drugs.)

Risk Factors Associated with Hyperlipaemia in the Donkey

Are you the owner of an over-weight jennet? - and aren't we all? If so, this article is for you.

Introduction

Hyperlipaemia is a life-threatening disease of ponies and donkeys (Jeffcott et al. 1986; Fowler 1989; Watson et al. 1992), in which the mortality rates are high. However, the report by Mair demonstrates that cases can be treated successfully. The metabolic disturbances underlying clinical signs are complex, involving plasma triglyceride concentrations, clearance of very low density lipoproteins (VLDL), lipoprotein lipase and insulin resistance. **The end result is multi-organ failure with deposition of lipid in liver and kidneys**.

Epidemiology of Hyperlipaemia

The epidemiology of the disease in the horse has recently been reviewed by Watson and Love (1994). Briefly, hyperlipaemia is a disease that occurs predominantly in mares, although occasionally males may be affected. In particular, in the female, it is associated with pregnancy and lactation (a time of major energy requirement) and this gives rise to the seasonal occurrence of cases.

Hyperlipaemia may be considered as either primary, where the only clinical signs are referable to hyperlipaemia or secondary, where prior or concurrent disease is diagnosed. The nature of the coexisting condition does not seem to be important with debility, inappetance, anorexia and endotoxaemia common features. Indeed, stress related to internal or external factors, disease or management, is a key feature in the history of affected animals. With specific reference to epidemiology in the donkey, less is known. Watson et al. (1992) demonstrated the relationship between body condition and plasma triglyceride and VLDL concentration with fat and obese animals having significantly higher concentrations of both analytes than donkeys at ideal weight. Similar to the horse, stress associated with environmental change and transport precipitates the disease.

In contrast to the specific knowledge gained from the individual sick donkey presented by Mair, population studies provide the opportunity to study the disease in more general terms. For diseases of low prevalence and incidence this is particularly important and because equids are usually kept in small groups, such opportunities arise infrequently.

Studies in the donkey

We have investigated hyperlipaemia in a population of over 4,000 donkeys and the results are providing new information on predisposing factors and survival of the hyperlipaemic crisis. The preliminary finds of this study presented recently used univariate and multivariate techniques in a study of 2 parts. First, the population records were screened for cases of hyperlipaemia and epidemiological factors associated with these animals compared to those of the non-hyperlipaemia population. Second, factors affecting survival of clinical hyperlipaemia were investigated in the case population.

Factors predisposing donkeys to hyperlipaemia

Several factors were found to be positively associated with the development of clinical hyperlipaemia. In common with previous reports, female animals were found to be more likely to get the disease than males. However, there were very few pregnant animals among the donkeys and no breeding occurs within the population thus providing evidence that aspects of female physiology, other than pregnancy and lactation are involved in predisposing jennies to the disease. *(Ed Note: I agree with the statement that female physiology predisposes jennets to the disease, however, my experience - and your phone calls - gives evidence to the fact the pregnancy and lactation (foaling) ways heavily in the onslaught of hyperlipaemia. Of all the phone calls I've received all but one jennet had foaled within 30 days of the diagnosis of hyperlipaemia and the one jennet was due to foal in one week.)*

Body condition was also a significant factor in the development of hyperlipaemia. The prevalence of the disease in **fat and obese** animals was higher than in animals in normal or thin condition. This finding supports the observation of Watson et al. Concerning the raised levels of VLDL and triglyceride in overweight donkeys. It was not possible to quantify the effect of concurrent disease in comparison to the non-hyperlipaemic population, 56% of cases were considered to be secondary to another disease process.

Donkeys also seemed to be more susceptible to developing hyperlipaemia at times of social and environmental stress. Changes of housing or mixing with a new group of animals leads to the establishment of new dominance hierarchies, an observation supported by the cases occurring after entry to the population.

Furthermore, animals that were younger (less than 10 years) at times of such stress were less likely to get the disease than older animals, perhaps due to the fact that younger animals are less prone to secondary disease or may be stronger and more successful in establishing dominance.

Factors affecting survival of the hyperlipaemic crisis

Animals that developed hyperlipaemia were divided into survivors and non-survivors and the epidemiological factors associated with each outcome group compared. In contrast to developing the disease, gender was not significantly associated with survival. Whether this would be true of a population where females were allowed to breed is open to debate because the severity of the disease may be exacerbated by the physiological stresses of gestation and abortion. (Ed Note: Again, we have determined that pregnancy is a significant factor.)

Overweight and obese animals were more likely to die than underweight donkeys, which in turn, were less likely to survive than donkeys of ideal weight. However, the most important factor influencing survival of hyperlipaemia ws the presence or absence of concurrent disease. In the multivariate analysis, the body condition of the animal was entered as either normal or abnormal, i.e., both over and underweight animals. Considered together, animals of normal body condition were approximately 7 times more likely to survive than fat and thin animals; donkeys with a concurrent disease were 8 times more likely to die than donkeys with primary hyperlipaemia.

Although stress during mixing and entry to the population may have been implicated in the precipitation of hyperlipaemia, survival of animals during this period was good. Close veterinary supervision identified cases early and instituted the appropriate therapeutic measures. The incidence of cases occurring at other times was low but these cases had poorer survival rates. On the whole, this seemed to be due to the fact that secondary hyperlipaemia was more common among these animals.

Conclusions

Despite the fact that the donkey with hyperlipaemia treated by Mair made a full recovery, there can be no doubt that the disease is frequently fatal. Even with the use of heparin and insulin therapy, 60% mortality rates may still be expected. Until such time as human lipid lowering drugs like nicotine acid, which inhibits lipolysis become available to the veterinarian practitioner, the emphasis must be on prevention rather than hope of a cure. To this end, the study reported briefly above provides preliminary points of action.

- Donkeys must be regarded as potential hyperlipaemia cases whenever they experience stress. This includes not only the time of socialization when mixing with new animals but also during transport and introduction to a new environment.
- Physiological stress due to obesity or malnutrition should be minimized by maintaining donkeys at a healthy body-weight. Care should be taken when attempting to control a donkey's weight so that food intake is not reduced to such a level that hyperlipaemia ensues.
- Female donkeys should be considered as high risk animals for hyperlipaemia even if they are not pregnant.
- Diseased donkeys should always be considered as potential cases of hyperlipaemia and attention paid to both primary disease and energy balance. Cases of hyperlipaemia secondary to other illnesses as illustrated by Mair are perhaps the most difficult to avoid. Certainly, inappetance precipitates the hyperlipaemic state and oral drenches of glucose in oral drenches or by i.v. infusion may be the only realistic methods of maintaining a positive energy balance.

The donkey, like man, is susceptible to stress. Attention to lifestyle and removal or prevention of identifiable stressors is important for the well being of both species. Whether it is artherosclerosis or hyperlipaemia, the consequences are all too frequently the same.

T.S. Mair Study

1. Hyperlipaemia is many times secondary to another disease.
2. Resting plasma trigylceride levels of normal donkeys are significantly higher than ponies and there is a positive correlation between levels of plasma free fatty acids/triglycerides and body condition of the donkeys. Recently, a positive correlation between plasma insulin and triglyceride concentrations was demonstrated in a group of donkeys with naturally occurring hyperlipaemia. Insensitivity to insulin appears, therefore, to be a major predisposing factor in the donkey.
3. Stressful conditions such as transportation, inclement weather or management changes act as common triggers for hyperlipaemia. A review of six cases of hyperlipaemia in donkeys treated by this author over the past 5 years revealved 2 cases associated with transportation and/or exposure to a new environment, one case associated with severe intestinal parasitism and 3 cases where there was no obvious causal factor.

The clinical features of hyperlipaemia are frequently vague and non-specific. Typical signs include depression, inappetance, weakness, muscle fasciculations, ataxia and reluctance to move. Intestinal motility and manure output are usually reduced and some animals may exhibit abdominal pain. Diarrhea was reported in some cases but this could reflect a primary intestinal disease rather than being associated with hyperlipaemia. Heart, respiratory rates and rectal temperature are often increased. Other clinical signs might include congested mucous membranes, jaundice halitosis and ventral oedema. After several days the condition deteriorates with anorexia, severe weight loss, neurological signs and eventually recumbency, convulsions and death.

Therapy of hyperlipaemia is designed to treat any underlying disease, correct and maintain energy balance and reduce plasma lipid concentrations. Treatments to correct and maintain energy balance are of the utmost importance. This author has found that enteral feeding of commercial preparations and slurries made of pelleted horse feeds' administered by nasogastric tube, is particularly useful.

(Ed Note: This next paragraph is rather technical but could be useful to your veterinarian if your donkey is diagnosed with hyperlipaemia.)

Treatment specifically to speed the removal of lipids from the blood are somewhat controversial. Insulin and glucose have been suggested to inhibit mobilization from adipose tissue, by inhibiting hormone sensitive lipase. Such treatment may predispose to lactic acidosis and to prevent this, alternative treatment of insulin combined with glucose and galactose on alternate days has been recommended. Because many affected animals appear to be insensitive to insulin, its therapeutic value is questionable. Haparin has been advocated for treatment by improving the clearance of plasma triglycerides via increase lipoprotein lipase activity. However, lipoprotein lipase activity is not defective in ponies with hyperlipaemia but is, rather, near maximum. Therefore, heparin administration is probably of small benefit. In man, heparin administration causes the serum to become less opaque, but this is due to an alteration of the chemical form of the lipid in the blood and total lipid content is unchanged. In addition, bleeding tendencies may be potentiated by heparin and it must be used with some caution.

In the absence of controlled studies that demonstration the effects of insulin and/or heparin therapy in clinical cases, benefits from these treatments remain uncertain. In this author's experience, prompt treatment of any underlying disease and provision of adequate nutritional support have proved to be the most effective therapies currently available for the treatment of hyperlipaemia in ponies and donkeys.

Reference: S.W.J. Reid and Sacha J. Cowan© Veterinary informatics and Epidemiology Group, Department of Veterinary Medicine, University of Glasgow Veterinary School, UK

Should you *Really* be using Ivomec® on your Donkeys?

(The answer is NO)

It has come to my attention that there are a number of breeders using Ivomec - cattle dewormer - on their donkeys.

I personally have purchased several donkeys over the years whose records indicated that they were "dewormed" with Ivomec. Most of the weanlings had rough, dull coats, large bellies, and were somewhat depressed. They did not act or play like weanlings their ages should. Upon arrival here, they were dewormed with either Zimecterin or Strongid equine paste dewormer. Normally within two weeks, their hair coats improved and they began to look and act healthier.

Several years ago, Ivomec developed an injectable equine dewormer. It was an oil base and veterinarians reported numerous severe abscesses at the injection sites, therefore the product was taken off the market.

Miniature Donkey Talk Magazine consulting veterinarians tell us that there have been no studies done on giving Ivomec cattle dewormer, orally to equine. Why? Because it was developed for cattle, ***not*** equine.

The insert that the distributor, Merch & Co,. puts inside each box of Ivomec states as follows: "Ivomec injection is indicated for the effective treatment and control of the following harmful species of gastrointestinal roundworms, lungworm, grubs, sucking lice and mange mites **in cattle.** **CAUTION:** Ivomec Injection for Cattle has been developed specifically for use in cattle and reindeer **ONLY**. This product should not be used in other animal species as severe adverse reactions, including fatalities in dogs, may result."

When the distributor warns against using this product on animals other than cattle and reindeer, why is it that some donkey breeders are using it? My number one guess is that they feel it is cost effective. Although a small bottle of dewormer cost around $32.00, it would last a very long time. Because of this, I also suspect that people are not paying attention to the expiration date on the bottle, making the product even more useless on donkeys.

Since my personal experience of purchasing donkeys who have been given Ivomec has been so negative, I am wondering the effectiveness of this drug on donkeys. If no studies have been done on the effectiveness of its use on equine parasites, my guess is that this drug is not effective on all parasites that are harmful to equine. With the numerous deworming products on the market specifically made for use in equine, why would anyone use a dewormer specifically made for cattle? If cost effectiveness is the reason, resulting veterinarian bills due to internal parasite damage will surely override the savings of using an ineffective dewormer.

Most equine dewormers state on their packaging whether they are safe for pregnant or very young equine. Some are not. Since Ivomec warns against using on any animals other than cattle and reindeer, who is foolish enough to risk using it on very young donkeys or bred jennets?

We advocate the use of equine dewormers ***only*** on your donkeys. There are numerous equine dewormers on the market which can readily be found in any part of the country.

Read your deworming paste labels carefully.

Safe-Guard and **Panacur** - Both safe for foals under the age of 4 months.
Zimecterin or **Eqvalan** are good for use between the months of December and March to rid your donkeys of bots. (Do not use on foals under 4 months of age.)
Strongid, Telmin B, Cutter are all good equine dewormers to use on adult donkeys.

Don't risk your donkeys very life on cheap deworming agents. It simply isn't worth it.

Chapter 11

Buying, Selling, Marketing

Why Miniature Donkeys?

by Bonnie Gross, Editor, Miniature Donkey Talk Magazine

There is no reason when thinking about Miniature Donkeys you can't have your cake and eat it too. When people call me and ask, "Why Miniature Donkeys?', my response is, "What other animal industry is there where you have a fantastic (and holding strong) investment combined with the ultimate pet"?

There are those out there who are making a living - and a good living - in the animal industry. These people have a wide variety of animals. When it comes to the animal industry as your sole means of support, the old saying, "Never put all your eggs in one basket", certainly comes into play. Those people on the other hand, are finding that Miniature Donkeys are making up a large portion of their incomes. The smaller breeder/investor is also finding donkeys to be a reliable and profitable source of second income.

Your initial investment and the desire to become a breeder, can be a heavy one. This ultimately brings several questions to mind. Is the market going to hold? Is this an industry that is hot today and gone tomorrow? How many years will it take me to recoup my investment? Are there tax advantages in this industry? What about the person with limited acreage?

Many animals who are hot one year are gone the next simply because the market has become saturated. These industries suddenly have drastic price increases for breeding stock and it seems everyone you know is breeding this particular animal. How much common sense does it take to realize that any animal that can produce in excess of 2, 3 or 4 offspring a year will soon flood the market. Once supply overrides demand, prices plummet. These other animals are also not the kind, loving and affectionate pets that Miniature Donkeys are.

Miniature Donkeys, on average, carry a foal for 12 months. Most are not rebred until their second heat cycle, some 30 odd days after foaling. Some jennets will not conceive until their foal is weaned. Taking all into consideration, the average jennet produces ONE offspring every 13 to 14 months. Considering the growing demand, it is highly unlikely - more like an impossibility - this market could become saturated.

How does the small breeder - the person looking for a second income - get started? How many donkeys are needed to produce a lucrative income? The small breeder obviously needs one breeding jack (male). Take for example that you bought one proven adult breeding jack at $2,500. Then you buy six adult breeding jennets at $2,500 to $4,500 each. Your initial outlay could be $24,000. Your first year your animals produce three jack foals @ $1,000 each and three jennet foals @ $2,500 each. Keep in mind we are talking typical gray-dun donkeys and not your more costly exotic colors. Your first year you could recoup close to 60% of your initial investment. Say lady luck is on your side and you produce six jennet foals (not all that difficult - We just had 8 jennets in a row born!). You could recoup near your entire investment in one year! There is also the obvious likelihood that in that group of six foals will be several of your more exotic colors, or ones with exceptional conformation or personality, which of course will sell for more.

Now I hear the rumbling of "where in the world am I going to get $24,000?" Every state has their own individual Farm Credit Bureaus which specialize in loaning money to farmers (large and small) for crops, equipment and livestock. Take with you a copy of *"MINIATURE DONKEY TALK"* Magazine and show them the ads. This will give you the proof in print of a viable investment.

Adding to your income, provided you set up your Miniature Donkey operation as a "business" and not as a "hobby", are federal income tax deduction allowances. You are allowed depreciation on your breeding stock along with deductions for feed, fencing, shelters, vet fees, advertising, insurance and other expenditures that are included in your operation. Also included would be the interest on your Farm Credit Loan!

Limited acreage can go hand in hand with Miniature Donkeys. You could easily keep 10 donkeys on an acre of land. This however doesn't mean they could live off pasture grasses. It does mean they could live comfortably being fed hay year round. You basically need a pasture large enough for them to run and play in to receive enough exercise for them to remain healthy.

I feel this industry is on a good platform at this time. It has proven itself with prices holding. Every specific animal industry has their breeders who do not know what the word *"reputation"* means and further more, probably don't care. Do your homework. Order all available back copies of *"MINIATURE DONKEY TALK"* Magazine and read and reread them - they contain a <u>wealth</u> of information. If you can't go visit several breeders, spend the money for the long distance phone calls. Have a list of questions in front of you. If you can visit breeders, take notice to their farms. Do the donkeys appear in good health? Are their hooves reasonably trimmed? Can the owners show you health records? What type of shelters do the donkeys have? Do you leave feeling that the breeder takes pride in their business? Are their donkeys underpriced?

Why? Are the donkeys of poor quality? No reputable breeder, who plans on staying in the business, will undercut their fellow breeders on quality animals. Are the donkeys overpriced? If so, are they of super quality or do you appear to be super gullible. A positive note that I do see in the classified ads in *MDT* is the beginning of breeders placing lower prices on lesser quality donkeys and/or donkeys they feel may not be top quality breeding stock for one reason or another. I feel this adds to the integrity of breeders and credence to the industry as a whole.

I keep a close eye on the other animal industries. I see a lot of fighting going on amongst the breeders. I do not however, see a lot of this within the Miniature Donkey industry. Take a look at *MDT's READER LETTERS* Section. At least every issue contains one letter stating ".....I just wanted to share", or "....I thought this may help other...". Sometimes I feel that the donkeys are not only a wonderful breed but also their owners are a wonderful breed! If when reading about Miniature Donkeys, you <u>only</u> have dollar signs in your eyes, you are probably not the compassionate animal lover that this industry needs and welcomes and would probably do better at another investment.

I have had several couples buy from me this year who have been getting *MDT* for in excess of one year. They've read, learned, listened and done their homework. They realize the Miniature Donkey industry remains on an upswing. They've made the investment and they've purchased the right animals. In all probability, they will have a successful and profitable business along with the joys and happiness the animal itself ultimately provides.

Buying Miniature Donkeys

With the rising popularity of Miniature Donkeys, many people call to ask what they should look for in buying them. Of course the first and foremost asked question is *"how much can I expect to pay for a Miniature Donkey?"* This is like asking how much you should pay for a car. Many things enter into the price put on a Miniature Donkey. Let's cover some of the aspects that will influence your choice in purchasing donkeys.

<u>Personality</u>

Are you looking simply for a pet? If so, personality should be your first concern. Most Miniature Donkeys are by nature very friendly and loving pets. They are extremely popular for senior citizens and families with small children. I have heard of very few aggressive or mean donkeys. The few I have heard of were breeding jacks who were brought up to be just that - breeding jacks and not pets. On the other hand, many letters in *MDT's Reader Letters Section* prove that many ungelded jacks have made excellent pets. I do not recommend that you buy an ungelded adult jack as a pet for a child. Even though the donkey's nature is to be much less nervous and tense than an ungelded horse, you cannot remove his basic instincts. You can buy an ungelded jack foal and at approximately one year of age, have him gelded making him safe around seniors and children. With regard to jennets, you may certainly come across "timid" ones. Most likely, they were not handled a lot as foals and are shy around people. These jennets will either run from people or crouch down and clamp their tail tightly against their bodies when approached. I have seen older jennets that ever after years of affectionate handling by their owners never change their timid behavior. Other jennets learn to trust people and will do a complete turn around within a matter of weeks. If you are buying a timid breeding jennet, her personality reflects on to the foal only to a certain point. For the first few days, you should handle her foal as much as possible. In a few days, you will then find that the foal will follow their mother's instincts and will also become timid around people. By the age of one month, simple curiosity takes over and foals want to investigate everything - including people. With handling you will find that they will become very friendly no matter how Mom feels about people. Again, it is important to handle them during their first few days of life to *imprint* your kindness on them and they will fall back on this.

Conformation

Are you looking for show or breeding animals? If so, then of course you want to avoid conformation faults. If you are only looking for a pet, a donkey with conformation faults will give you just as much love and affection as a show quality one will.

Every breeder has their own idea of what they want to breed for. This is their privilege and their right as a breeder. However, I think most breeders agree that Miniature Donkeys should give the first impression of being small and compact with a drafty type look to them. Miniature Donkeys were originally a working breed. A miniature with long, thin legs and a petite body - although pretty to look at - would not be a good working animal.

Most people don't realize just how very important the conformation of their breeding jack is. ***MDT*** sent out a survey and the consensus among most breeders is that a jack can determine 75% of the conformation of the foal. Not all jacks carry this strong conformation gene, however, if you desire to begin a breeding operation, your jack should be your most important purchase! When looking at breeding age jennets, *smaller is not necessarily better!* You want to keep your breeding jennets between the sizes of 32" to 36" and a breeding jack 30" to 33". The original donkeys brought into this country by the August Busch Family (of Busch Beer fame) were between the sizes of 32" and 38". Jennets under the height of 32" tend to have foaling (birthing) problems. When looking at breeding age jennets, you must keep in mind that with each foal, more of her "girlish" figure disappears. Older jennets may have somewhat of a sway back and stretched stomach muscles. What you might think are conformation defects may in fact be the result of the birth of several foals.

Two serious conformation defects you want to avoid when buying donkeys you intend to use for breeding purposes are parrot mouth, monkey mouth and cow-hocks. Parrot and monkey mouths are where the top or bottom teeth protrude out further than 1/4" from the opposite set of teeth. As an added note, I have personally looked into the mouths of hundreds of donkeys and can honestly say that the majority of donkeys have slight over or underbites of 1/16 to 1/4 inch. Registered or Unregistered?? Some Miniature Donkey Registrys are based on size only. The **International Miniature Donkey Registry** in Westminster, Maryland is a graded registry. You would be wise to make sure your intended purchase carries IMDR registration papers. Inspect your intended purchases closely, check their teeth and conformation, and make your decisions based on the quality of each individual animal.

Many donkeys stand slightly cowhocked. You simply cannot compare the stature of a donkey to a horse and will do a donkey injustice if you do so. Severely cowhocked hind legs is a definite conformation defect and these donkeys should be avoided when you are purchasing show or breeding stock.

Color

The most prevalent color for Miniature Donkeys is gray-dun which consists of a gray colored body, light colored nose - or dark colored nose -, light colored belly and inside legs, with a dark color dorsal stripe down the back and over the shoulders. The dorsal stripe is known as the donkeys cross. Colors other than the typical gray-dun makes the donkey more exotic looking therefore increases their price. There are different colors of sorrel, various colors of brown, spotted colors of donkeys (usually white and gray) and a very limited number of true blacks, whites and albino.

Age

When buying Miniature Donkeys, you will normally pay a little less for foals than you would for breeding age donkeys, unless the foal is of an exotic color, pedigree or has outstanding conformation. Jennet foals command much higher prices than do jack foals. Most people ask why and the reasoning is very simple. One breeding jack can service many breeding jennets. With life long proper care, donkeys can live well into their 30's and jennets can produce foals into their 20's. Older jennets are normally wonderful mothers and fantastic baby sitters to put in with foals being weaned.

Height

Desirable heights of Miniature Donkeys will vary with almost every person you talk to. The best I can do here is to give you my personal opinion. I suggest that people purchase jennets to be used for breeding be between the height of 32" to 36". Jennets in this size range tend to have better conformation and an easier time of foaling than do smaller jennets. Smaller jennets normally need some assistance in delivering a foal. If that assistance is not at hand, you take the chance of losing the foal and possibly the mother. When buying jacks, again pay particular attention to conformation first, size second. Here at *Pheasant Meadow Farm* we have several sets of three generations: Grandmother, Mother and Daughter. I can assure you that Grandparents can play a large role in the conformation, coloring and height of a foal.

Where To Buy Miniature Donkeys

Before buying any breed of animal you should do your homework and have an idea of what you are looking for. Breeders who advertise in *"MINIATURE DONKEY TALK"* Magazine will be happy to talk to you and share with you their experiences in raising and breeding Miniature Donkeys. We encourage you to contact us at *"MINIATURE DONKEY TALK"* or any of our advertisers to help you with your questions. If you are buying your first Miniature Donkey, you definitely want to buy from a reputable breeder located anywhere within the U.S. or Canada as donkeys are currently being shipped at great distances. Make certain you use a reputable horse transportation company and ask them for references. Miniature Donkeys are also sold at exotic animal auctions however, if you are new to the donkey world, we definitely suggest that you take an experienced owner with you.

Shipping Donkeys

Many of you make contact with a reputable breeder who has donkeys for sale, but they always seem to be on the other side of the earth. Considering the purchase price of donkeys, shipping costs are rather reasonable. We use an excellent equine trucking company to do our shipping. Below are some prices we have paid on donkeys being shipped from Baltimore, Maryland to the following locations: Kansas (1 donkey) $465; Georgia (4 donkeys) $620; Kentucky (3 donkeys) $475; California (2 donkeys) $875; North Washington State (3 donkeys) $1325; Wisconsin (1 donkey) $325; Minnesota (2 donkeys) $425; Missouri (2 donkeys) $350; Colorado (2 donkeys) $575; New York (2 donkeys) $200, Washington State (2 weanlings) $975. Prices are generally quoted on a 35 cent to 50 cent per mile basis depending on destination.

You are normally charged by the "stall area". One large horse fits into one stall area. Two donkey foals, yearlings or two smaller adults can fit into one stall area. We do not personally like to air freight donkeys however some people do. This is usually limited to weanlings. There are minimum and maximum air temperature requirements, they must fly into and out of a large international airport and there have been problems with flights being canceled and shipping crates being too small. We suggest that you investigate shipping by air and make your own decisions.

Cold Weather Care

"Donkeys are made to be Donkeys"

Here we go again: we're about to be zapped by the nasty weather, and with it comes the perennial crop of well-intentioned concerns when it comes to looking after our donkeys. Although these are spawned by a sincere desire to do right by our donkeys, nevertheless, we so often fail to recognize the resilience and hardiness of most donkeys.

All too often, the solutions that we think are correct are misguided; whereas the ones that treat donkeys like donkeys are most sound.

"My donkey is getting thin, I'd better increase the grain ration."

Most adult donkeys do fine without any grain at all. Instead, you should take an honest look at your hay ration and your deworming program. Are you really feeding enough quality hay? Many parts of the U.S. had more than normal amounts of rain this past summer, and others had draught, but now the grass is not growing or is of much lower quality. If your donkey is scrounging around picking up every last piece of hay, you need to reevaluate how much your are feeding. Roughage is the foundation of your donkey's diet. If your donkeys are not properly dewormed, the worms will definitely rob your animal of needed nutrients.

"Looks like rain or snow is on the way. I'd better keep the donkeys locked in the barn."

Your donkeys should be turned out every day. We have a large barn and our donkeys and horses come and go at will. The barn is always open for them. We have a board nailed across the donkey entrance so the large horses cannot get into the donkey's part of the barn. Since we have a slight hill in front of the barn, the only time we lock up the donkeys and horses is during a ice storm as the ground is treacherous. Donkeys are outdoor animals and need to be able to get out and interact with each other. It is proven that donkeys and horses who have barns and run-in sheds, that they can leave and enter at will, have much lower incidence of respiratory disease. We once had a jennet experience very painful gas colic from staying in the barn and not moving around enough.

"It's going to get cold tonight, I think I'll put a blanket on my donkey."

Unclipped, healthy donkeys do much better without a blanket as their coats have natural insulation abilities. Blankets mash down the coat and can actually chill a donkey. The only exception may be freezing rain and/or a very cold wind storm. If you are new to donkeys, you may not realize how thick their winter coats are. When they start to shed out in the spring, you'll understand what I mean...

"It's going to be so cold tonight I'd better make sure all the windows and doors are closed on the barn."

Nothing is worse for a donkey than a barn with no ventilation. Stale air and ammonia fumes can invade a donkey's defenses to fight off bacteria and viruses. In an air tight barn, one donkey harboring a slight respiratory virus can quickly spread it to everyone else. If you have a wind slamming against one side of the barn, leave the opposite side of the barn open.

"I'd better check up on my donkey's flu vaccination and make sure

he's up to date."

Flu shots are fine but how about that rhino vaccination? Equine herpes virus (EHV) also known as rhinopneumonitis, also known as rhino can be just as deadly if not more so as it pertains to donkeys. Most people just simply call an upper respiratory outbreak the flu when clinical findings may very well indicate that it is rhino. A lot of vaccinations come in 4-way and 5-way and don't include rhino because it has to be given separately, many people think they are fully vaccinating their donkey. We find donkeys to be just as susceptible to rhino as they are flu so do not forget that very important rhino vaccination. And don't forget deworming. A donkey stressed out due to worms has a much greater chance of dying from a severe respiratory illness.

"It's a cold one today, think I'll give my donks a big scoop of grain to keep them warm."

Wrong! Grain provides very little heat to the donkey if any, and this includes corn. Hay keeps the donkey warm because fermenting digestion of the hay generates caloric heat. Donkeys are designed to eat a little, all day long. Feeding good quality hay will keep your donkey warm, over a longer period of time, plus provides plenty of fiber which is important to keep the intestinal tract functioning properly.

"I've chipped off the top layer of ice so the donkeys have water to drink."

Chipping away ice may not be enough. Warming the water to a drinkable temperature has shown to significantly increase consumption. A dehydrated donkey is not digesting its food properly and is very prone to colic and other digestive problems. We have automatic waterers that have a heating element in them that keeps the water in winter at about 45 degrees. If you do not have this luxury (that's what I consider it if you aren't forced to haul heavy buckets of water!) then you need to haul hot water to poor over the ice. There are all kinds of electrical ice melting gadgets out there. Check the wiring often and be careful not to get the water too hot and burn the donkey.

Use your good judgment in caring for your donkeys in winter weather. A happy donkey is usually a healthy donkey.

Reference: Written by Bonnie Gross, *Editor, MDT Magazine*

Marketing Miniature Donkeys

There are probably as many marketing strategies as there are people to market this nice animals. Each seller has to arrive at an individual style of marketing that best suits their philosophical outlook, personality and the financial necessity to make a sale. Marketing is defined as the act of promoting, cultivating a clientele for, and selling any good or service.

Who Buys Miniature Donkeys

It seems important that we determine who is buying what we are selling. Essentially there appears to be two broad types of buyers for Miniature Donkeys. The first are people interested in deriving an income from breeding and selling Miniature Donkeys. The second are people interested in purchasing a unique, fairly rare backyard pet or companion. The backgrounds of these buyers are varied as some have owned horses in the past, some have owned other types of livestock and still others have never owned any type of livestock but the diminutive size of the donkey appeals to them more than a 16 hand horse would. The initial purchase is probably the result of simply the desire to own a unique little animal.

Miniature donkeys are not a necessity of life such as housing, food and clothing. They are a luxury item frequently purchased with money from savings accounts. The money may well have been spent on boats, vacations and other luxuries. Prevailing economic attitudes can heavily effect the sale of Miniature Donkeys. It is important that the seller be aware of current trends in the economy in order to determine the direction of emphasis for his or her marketing strategy.

It would be interesting to know how often buyers sell close to home and how often they sell outside their area. We at *Pheasant Meadow Farm* rarely sell close to home as the majority of our buyers are other breeders in the midwest or west coast as there are few breeders on the east coast. However, from all the people we talk to and correspond with, we feel that at this time, most sales take place between breeders and first time buyers and not breeders to breeders. If this assumption is correct, the market is healthy due to this new interest. There are buyers for every Miniature Donkey. The key is to bring the buyer and donkey together.

A highly positive aspect of marketing Miniature Donkeys is their appeal. Most people are genuinely taken with their small size, the cute fuzzy look of weanlings and overly friendly personalities.

Establishing a Price

Probably the biggest determiner as to whether a buyer is going to seriously consider your donkey is your asking price. Any price you put on a donkey can be the right price if you have a buyer who is willing to pay it. Potential buyers of donkeys are no different than buyers of other items. The educated buyer is going to do some comparison shopping. Each buyer has criteria that must be met before they purchase and a sale depends on whether your donkey meets this criteria. The *first time buyer* may have some of these factors in mind: By the way, these are not listed in any priority.

1. Personality - Another breeder may just be looking for good breeding stock and not be overly interested in how friendly the donkey is. Personality is almost always at the top of the list for first time buyers because in donkeys, this is what has attracted them in the first place.
2. Height - We often find this to be at the bottom of the list. First time buyers looking for pets are generally not concerned with height.
3. Sex - On average, jennets command higher prices than jacks unless the jack is outstanding in some way.
4. Pedigree - We find that donkeys sired by well-known, well-advertised herd sires command higher prices.
5. Conformation - Although extremely important for breeding stock, we find that many first time buyers do not learn about conformation strengths and weaknesses until after they purchase their first donkeys. This is unfortunate as we often get calls from these people saying, "The first donkeys I bought did not have very good conformation and now I'm looking for good stock."
6. Show record - With the limited number of shows around, we find this to be a non-issue with new buyers.
7. Age - New buyers generally have their minds made up as to whether they are looking for weanlings, adults or older breeder stock. We are fortunate that donkeys have a long life span so even those in their teens are still marketable.

Other factors affecting the price of the donkey can be the sellers personal situation. How anxious are you to sell? The higher the price, the fewer qualified buyers available. One needs to keep in mind that the price will reflect how fast the donkey sells. The lower the price the more buyers there are available.

The sellers emotional bond to the donkey will also reflect on the price set. Being attached to a donkey doesn't mean that potential buyers will see the same qualities in the donkey as you do.

When setting a price you need to put emotion and biases away and honestly evaluate the animal. A seller can ask as much as he wants for the donkey, but its true worth at any particular time is measured by what a buyer is willing to pay.

Exposure to the public

The more your business and farm is exposed to the public, the more sales you'll have. Most advertisers in *Miniature Donkey Talk Magazine* sell donkeys with ease. Repetitive advertising keeps your name and your farm in plain view and easy to recognize. New buyers feel more comfortable buying from sellers who take the time and expense to promote their donkeys. They feel more at ease in asking questions and feel repeat advertisers will be around if months down the road they have questions. We find that new buyers especially like to have weanlings from well known herd sires.

Buyers interested in breeding Miniature Donkeys and selling their offspring need to not only spend the money to purchase quality donkeys, they need to have money set aside for advertising on a continual basis. So many first time buyers feel that when its time for them to sell, people will automatically come to their door. If you aren't willing to take the time and effort to promote yourself and your donkeys, then you need to realize you'll have to accept lower prices for your donkeys.

"Twenty percent of the sellers make eighty percent of the sales and the other eighty percent of the sellers divide the remaining twenty percent of the sales." The more often people see your advertising in *Miniature Donkey Talk*, the more name recognition you have. You of course need to base your advertising on what you expect to have in future sales. If you are producing one or two foals a year, then running a full page color ad for a year seems rather silly. On the other hand, if you have high quality stock, producing high quality offspring there is no better way to show off your animals than with a glossy color ad. For smaller breeders producing limited numbers, a business card ad may be all that's needed to keep your name out in public and develop name recognition.

Low Cost Exposure
There are a variety of lost cost ways to promote your animals locally.

Participate in parades
Attend county fairs
Take your donkeys to public facilities like nursing homes, schools.
Contact your chamber of commerce and let them know you may be open for tours.
Shopping mall openings

Making an Impression

Try to remember what is was the impressed you the most with the people you bought your first donkey from. Was it their advertising? The cleanliness of their facilities? Their personalities? The quality of their donkeys? The odd thing about a lot of new buyers is that they are impressed by things that many times do not even reflect on the quality of the animal they are buying.

The first impression of your farm is something that many buyers always remember. Many other buyers are only concerned with the immediate area that the donkeys are in. If buyers are distracted by smell, mud and poor facilities, it will be hard for them to concentrate on evaluating the donkey.

Physical condition of the donkey

Even inexperienced buyers seem to be able to pick up on the fact that a donkey is not healthy. Poor coat quality and thin animals reflect badly on your entire herd and your management practices. If you are selling during wet weather, try to clean the donkey up and keep it clean before the buyer arrives. If you are selling in winter, please think of the welfare of the donkey before you decide to body clip it. Nothing turns new buyers off faster than long untrimmed hooves.

Well kept records

You should be able to tell potential buyers all about vaccinations and dewormings on the donkey you have for sale. If the animal is an adult, you should know in advance all the foals produced and should be able to answer any health questions relating to the animal. Buyers do not like to hear "all the donkeys were vaccinated last year" because they don't believe you. They want dates. They want to know that you are going to give them all health records in writing when they pick the donkey up.

Selling yourself

We all live busy lives these days. Buyers and/or browsers should not show up without appointments and if they do, they need to expect that you may very well not have time for them. On the other hand, if appointments are made, expect to spend as much time with the buyer as the buyer wants. Open yourself up for all the questions that they want to ask and invite those questions. If something rotten in going on in your life, mention a little of it to your visitors or simply tell them that you're having a rotten day. Don't let them walk away feeling like they intruded on you or they were not welcomed when it wasn't that at all. Encourage questions and be forthcoming with information. Ask potential buyers about their farm and try to get a feel of what type of donkeys would best fit their needs.

Written or telephone inquiries

You receive one of those letters asking about your donkeys or what you have for sale. You get a phone call asking if you have information you can send out. Are these people tire-kickers or are they serious buyers. Who knows? That is why you have to take the time to answer their requests. Even if you do not have what they are looking for at the moment, they might not be ready to buy now but are gathering information so when they are ready, they'll come visit you. I have a general information packet covering donkeys in both general terms and also in more detail. It not only covers the glory aspects of owning donkeys but gives buyers details on the work involved properly caring for livestock. I want potential buyers to know in advance that animal ownership is not all fun and games. However you respond to written inquires, you should remember that they are also writing other farms and your written information will be in competition with others.

The FF's - Friendly Foals

Nothing appeals more to potential buyers than fuzzy little foals running up to them begging for attention. What gives the better impression: 1) foals running up, pulling on pant legs, untying shoe laces and rubbing against legs, or, 2) you out there, waving arms, herding up a group into a small corral so you can get near them. It takes very little effort on your part having foals that are overly friendly. Spending time with them, scratching and rubbing, during their first week of life guarantees an appealing very saleable pet.

Your share of the market

No matter what business you are in there is always some form of competition. An important part of marketing is the manner in which the producer cultivates his share of the market. People remain in business because of the strategy they use in attracting buyers. Here are some of the strategies people use in carving out a share of the marketplace.

1. Breeding for a specific color.
2. Breeding for small size.
3. Breeding for conformation, regardless of color
4. Breeding lots of different types of donkeys for good selection.
5. Dealers who do very little breeding but more buying and reselling.

One thing to keep in mind if you get too specialized is that you greatly limit your clientele. Many times your specialty will depend on the size of your herd.

Unfortunately there are a number of highly questionable practices employed to 'get in on the action'. These people are selling donkeys to make money, period. The sad thing is that less than ethical business practices reflects on the rest of us who work so hard. We've heard so many new buyers becoming disenchanted after being sold donkeys that were misrepresented. Educating naïve buyers as to the potential pitfalls in buying can be an excellent marketing tool. Buyers appreciate the guidance.

I highly encourage all potential buyers to visit as many farms as possible before buying. I ask that they become as educated as they possibly can on evaluating conformation. When they are ready to buy, but do not have the money to buy top of the line, at least they know what they are buying and will not feel taken advantage of. Some times buyers simply want back yard pets and have no interest in breeding therefore have no desire or need for top quality breeding stock. Any breeder who tells potential buyers that they always have top quality foals has either not been in business long, has not had many foals, or simply has no understanding of donkey conformation. No matter how great your breeding stock, pet quality foals are going to pop out from time to time. Buyers understand this. Do not insult their intelligence by claiming otherwise.

Word of mouth

One of the most powerful marketing tools is word of mouth recommendations from other breeders or people who have purchased from you. Several breeders can work together so if a buyer comes to one and the breeder doesn't have what they are looking for, they can refer them to another farm. We find that when we refer someone to another breeder and they are treated fairly, the buyer still comes back to us when they are ready to purchase more donkeys. Of course you need to make sure that the seller you are referring the buyer to is reputable or the referring farm can suffer a loss of credibility. A solid reputation, gained by your fairness in doing business is like money in the bank.

Rated Registrations

The *International Miniature Donkey Registry* developed a wonderful conformation rating system. Ratings were designed to help new or inexperienced buyers in determining well-conformed donkeys without having to know a lot about conformation. They can buy with the knowledge that some independent party has reviewed this donkey and has given an evaluation of the animal. Rating reviews also help breeders in their breeding programs. Evaluations help by pointing out certain faults that may be overcome by proper matching of breeding pairs, and producing better conformed foals. Ratings also help justify your asking price versus someone selling unregistered or non rated donkeys. Many buyers call IMDR and ask to be referred to breeders who have rated their donkeys which gives buyers a big advantage in purchasing quality animals. Ratings are a wonderful tool for both the buyer and the seller!

Marketing strategies can be very spartan endeavors or can run the gambit all the way to large scale promotional plans. Developing your approach to marketing your donkeys is a very important step and should be well thought out. Reference: Written by Bonnie Gross, *Editor, MDT Magazine*

Most Commonly Asked Questions from New Owners

1. *Why is my foal eating Mom's manure?*

This is nature's way of introducing bacteria into the intestines of the newborn. It's perfectly normal.

2. *Can I feed grass clippings to my donkeys?*

It's a dangerous practice. There are many poisonous ornamental shrubs that people have in their lawns and a very small amount can kill a donkey.

3. *Can my jennet be bred when she's 1-1/2 years old?*

You NEVER want to breed before the age of two years. If you do, the chances are very good the mother will reject the foal completely and/or she will abort mid-term because she is not mature enough herself to produce a viable foal. Waiting until a jennet is 2-1/2 to 3 years of age is best.

4. *When do jacks start breeding?*

Most jacks start their breeding careers between 16 and 19 months of age. Every jack is an individual. Our jack produced his first foal when he was a yearling. Other jacks we've had did not produce their first foal until they were 2 years old.

5. *What is the average gestation for a jennet?*

Average is 11 months, 3 weeks.

6. *If I geld my jack, can I keep him in with my jennets?*

Again, this all depends on the individual jack. Some jacks even after being gelded persist in harassing jennets. Other jacks lose all sexual desires and it works out great.

7. *Can I put my new weanling in with my very laid back horse?*

Sure. Some times it takes a few days for the horse to get used to the sight on this other 'strange looking equine' but we've had our donkeys in with horses for years.

8. *How much land do I need to keep a donkey on?*

Donkeys should have a minimum of one acre of land. They need room to run and play and exercise. They also need shelter - preferably a darken barn in summer to get away from biting flies. One acre of land will not meet their nutritional requirements of course so you would need to feed them hay year 'round. You also need to check your zoning laws. Donkeys are livestock. Some localities require 3 acres for livestock, others one acre and still others 5 acres.

9. *Can donkeys be housebroken*?

No. Of course there may be a handful of people on this earth who claim they have a housebroken donkey and if you look hard enough, you may just find one that really is. Use your common sense here. Again, donkeys are livestock. How many housebroken horses have you heard of? How many housebroken cows? Goats? If you give it some thought, the concept of attempting to housebreak livestock is a silly one and should not be given serious thought.

10. *Will donkeys get along with my dogs*?

90% of all donkeys have a dislike of dogs. Most seem to really detest small dogs. HOWEVER, many many people who have donkeys also have dogs and if breeders raise newborn donkeys around dogs, there's an excellent chance that they can get along nicely. Mothers with foals can never be trusted around dogs even if they got along with them before they had their foal, simply because new mothers are so protective. My pastures that surround my yard are 4-board fencing and because we have small dogs, we lined the bottom of the fence with small gauge wire so that the dogs cannot get in the pastures, so there IS a workable solution.

11. *Can you put donkeys in with horses*?

Yes. Most of my donkeys are pastured with two horses. My gelding horse adores the donkeys and his greatest thrill is to lick a newborn donkey foal! The other horse is a mare and she would be happy never to see a donkey again. She would not hurt a donkey, but the donkeys know to give her plenty of room and to avoid close contact with her. Generally, donkeys and horses get along fine. Our barn is left open 24 hours a day so the donkeys and horses can enter and leave the barn at will. The donkey's section of the barn is cordoned off so that the horses cannot enter their section.

12. *Will donkeys get along with my goats*?

Sometimes. It has come to my attention over the years that a few breeders like to tell people that young jacks (males) make great companions for goats. FALSE! An ungelded young jack should never be pastured with goats. The main problem seems to be that young jacks like to play with goats the same way they play with each other - by grabbing the goat by the necks with their teeth. I lost count of how many phone calls I've gotten from grieving goat owners telling me how they found their goats dead from a broken neck. As a young jack comes of age, play turns to sexual aggression and the problem is worsened. So, can jennets (females) be pastured with goats? Possibly. Jennets do not play as aggressively as jacks so the chances of a jennet being pastured with goats has a better chance of working out. Some owners have told me that they give their goats an 'escape route' so if a jennet decides to play with or chase the goats, they can jump up on a large wooden box or have a small entrance into a separate barn that the donkey cannot get through.

13. *Can I buy just one donkey*?

Donkeys are herd animals. They love being with other donkeys. I personally will not sell one donkey to a person who has no other livestock. A lone donkey is a lonely donkey, a lonely donkey can be a stressed-out donkey, and a stressed-out donkey can end up being a sick donkey. It's always best to have two donkeys. They'll develop an extremely close friendship that will do your heart good.

14. *Do I need a barn for my donkey*?

Yes, in summer donkeys need a dark barn to get away from biting flies. In winter, donkeys need a place to get out of the weather. Most donkeys hate rain and snow and need appropriate shelter depending on where you live.

15. *Can I feed my donkey treats*?

Yes, but NEVER feed them by hand. This encourages biting fingers as donkeys will always be looking for a hand out. Put the treat on a clean clump of grass or in a feed pan. Some treats are bread, crackers, rolls, carrots, apples.

16. *Can donkeys pull carts and wagons*?

They sure can! Many many people train them to pull carts and have loads of fun with them. We have a large chapter in our book, *Caring For Your Miniature Donkey,* that begins at step one on training your donkey, buying tack and so on.

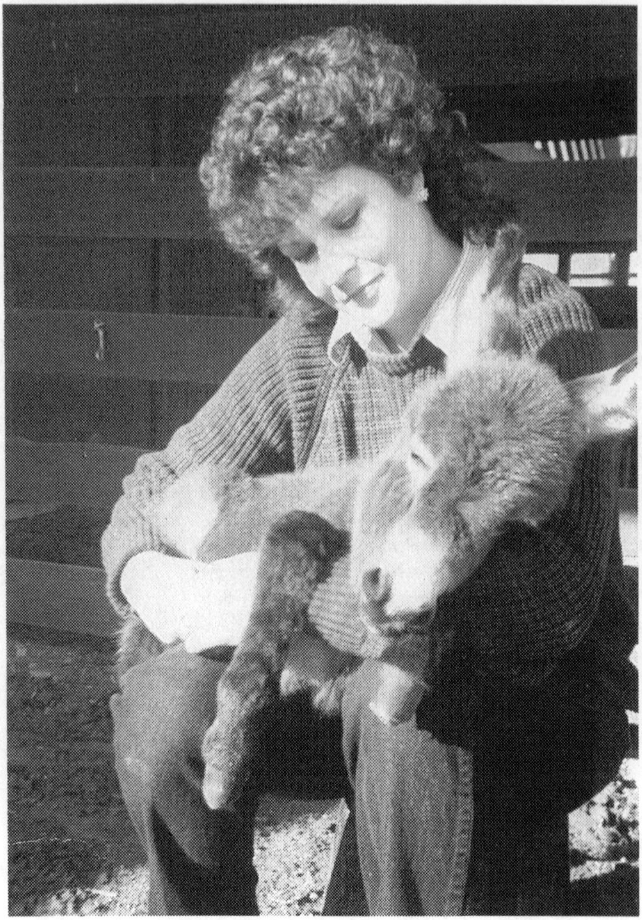

Bonnie Gross

I. M. D. R.

INTERNATIONAL MINIATURE DONKEY REGISTRY, Inc.

The official Miniature Donkey Registry for today and the future.

For Miniature Donkeys 38" and under
Size Classification:
Class A: 36" and Under
Class B: 36.1" to 38"

Five easy steps to apply for Registration: You do not have to be a member of IMDR to register a donkey, however the registration fees are more expensive if you are not a member. See fee schedules below.

1. Call IMDR for Registration Applications.
2. Take pictures. The registry needs two photos of the left side, and two of the right side. These may be duplicates. One set goes on the back of the regisration certificate and the other set goes on file with the application. Take photographs in good light so all identifyable marks can be recognized.
3. Fill out the application form and all pedigree information. Pedigrees are not required for registration, but if they are known they should be indicated.
4. Complete the owner and breeder information on the form exactly as you want it to show on all registration certificates.
5. Enclose all with appropriate fees by check or enclosed credit card information.

IMDR Membership Information One Year Renewable Membership: $18.00
Five Year Renewable Membership: $70.00
Special Lifetime Memberships (reduced registration fees) are available on request.

Registrations and Transfer Fees: **Permanent**: Over 2 years of age $18 member; $22 non-member; **Temporary**: Under 2 years of age $12.50 member; $15 non-member
Pet or Gelding: $8 member; $10 non-member
Transfer from any other registry to IMDR: $10

Special IMDR Rating Program: IMDR has a special donkey rating program. This computer generated conformation grading system is unique and of great help to new buyers. When considering buying an adult donkey with IMDR registration papers, ask the seller what the IMDR Rating is on the donkey. Ratings are based strictly on conformation. A Two, Three or Four Star rating means that you are purchasing a quality animal. Write IMDR for details.

1338 Hughes Shop Rd Westminster, MD 21158
Tel 410-875-0118 24 Hr Fax 410-857-9145
(Office Hours 9AM-4PM EASTERN STANDARD TIME Mon-Fri)

INDEX

Claude
Brockett
Donkey Hdq.
Box 1
Grandview, TX 76050